TELENEUROLOGY

TELENEUROLOGY

Complete Guide to Implementing Telemedicine and Telebehavioral Health into Your Practice

Edited by

RANDALL WRIGHT, MD

Director of the Brain Wellness and Sleep Program,
Houston Methodist Hospital,
The Woodlands, TX, United States

Clinical Faculty EnMed, Texas A&M University
College of Medicine, College of Engineering, Houston,
TX, United States

ELSEVIER

Elsevier
1600 John F. Kennedy Blvd.
Ste 1800
Philadelphia, PA 19103-2899

Notice

Practitioners and researchers must always rely on their own experience and knowledge in evaluating and using any information, methods, compounds or experiments described herein. Because of rapid advances in the medical sciences, in particular, independent verification of diagnoses and drug dosages should be made. To the fullest extent of the law, no responsibility is assumed by Elsevier, authors, editors or contributors for any injury and/or damage to persons or property as a matter of products liability, negligence or otherwise, or from any use or operation of any methods, products, instructions, or ideas contained in the material herein.

Library of Congress Control Number: 2021937494

Publisher: Cathy Sether
Acquisitions Editor: Melanie Tucker
Editorial Project Manager: Kristi Anderson
Production Project Manager: Poulouse Joseph
Cover Designer: Christian Bilbow

Printed in India.

Last digit is the print number: 9 8 7 6 5 4 3 2 1

Working together
to grow libraries in
developing countries

www.elsevier.com • www.bookaid.org

Contents

Video contents   *xi*
Contributors   *xiii*
About the editor   *xv*
Introduction   *xvii*
  Stanley H. Appel, MD

1. Responding to a crisis: A call to action   **1**
  Stephen Spielman, MBA, MHA

  Introduction   1
  Virtual foundation   1
  COVID-19   3
  Training   4
  Communication   5
  Virtual urgent care   6
  Patient feedback   6
  Physician feedback   7
  Conclusion   10

2. The telemedicine exam general overview   **11**
  Randall Wright, MD, Ronald Goldsberry

  The virtual visit   13
  Technical aspects of the virtual visit   16
  References   20

3. The TeleStroke evaluation   **21**
  Nhu Bruce, MD

4. Telemedicine for evaluation of clinical epilepsy   **25**
  Katherine Noe, MD, PhD

  Introduction   25
  Opportunities in virtual epilepsy care   25
  Initial epilepsy history and physical examination   26
  Evaluation and ongoing management   27
  Summary   29
  References   29

5. **The ophthalmologic exam**   **31**
    Garvin Davis, MD, MPH

    Introduction   31
    Patient selection   31
    Scheduling visits   31
    Software and hardware technology solutions   32
    The traditional ophthalmic exam   32
    Visual acuity   33
    Pupil exam   35
    Ocular motility   36
    Visual field   36
    Intraocular pressure   36
    External exam (eyelids and globe position in the orbit)   36
    Anterior segment exam   36
    Fundus or retina exam   36
    The hybrid telemedicine model   37
    Home monitoring   37
    Conclusion   37
    References   37

6. **Neuro-ophthalmology evaluation**   **39**
    Stacy V. Smith, MD

    Introduction   39
    Preparing for a telehealth visit   39
    The virtual visit   41
    Conclusion   44
    References   45

7. **Teleneurology for Parkinson's disease and movement disorders
    in the COVID-19 pandemic**   **47**
    Zoltan Mari, MD, FAAN

    Introduction   47
    Telemedicine in your movement disorder practice   49
    Conclusions   54
    References   54

8. **Introduction to tele-psychology during the pandemic**   **57**
    Annette E. Brissett, PhD

9. Tele-neuropsychology: Bringing neuropsychology into the
    future of health care delivery   61
    Kenneth Podell, PhD

    Patient satisfaction   63
    Research in tele-neuropsychology   64
    Tele-NP models   66
    "Connecting" with the patient   68
    Improving clinical outcomes   68
    Improving tele-NP visits   69
    Consent form   69
    Neuropsychological reports   72
    Billing tele-NP   73
    Interstate practice   74
    Future of tele-NP   75
    Resources   76
    Summary   77
    References   77

10. Sleep telemedicine   81
     Pablo R. Castillo, MD

     Overview   81
     Sleep telemedicine diagnostic approaches   81
     Sleep telemedicine treatment approaches   85
     Telemedicine follow-up approaches   85
     Conclusion   86
     References   87

11. Neuromuscular evaluation   89
     Ericka Greene, MD

     The history of telemedicine   89
     Telemedicine in neurology   89
     Telemedicine in neuromuscular disease   90
     Telemedicine in neurology in the COVID-19 era   94
     Telemedicine in neuromuscular medicine in the COVID-19 era   95
     Conclusion   101
     References   102

12. General neurosurgery exam   **105**
Jonathan J. Lee, MD, Gavin W. Britz, MD, MPH, MBA, FAANS

Introduction   105
Introductory interview questions   105
Mental status   106
Cranial nerve exam   109
Strength exam   111
The Babinski reflex   112
Sensory exam   113
Coordination   113
Conclusions   114
References   114

**13. Neurosurgical spine care during COVID-19 pandemic:
The Department of Neurological Surgery Houston
Methodist experience**   **117**
Fernando E. Silva, MD, Gavin W. Britz, MD, MPH, MBA, FAANS,
Paul Holman, MD

Introduction   117
Our approach   117
The visit   118
Evaluation/examination   118
Diagnosis   120
Treatment   121
Limits of telemedicine   122
Conclusion   122
References   123

14. System coordination and implementation   **125**
John J. Volpi, MD

Core values should guide decisions   127
Case 1: Dr. Garcia needs help at the hospital   127
Discussion   129
Solutions and realignment   129
Takeaways   130
Case 2: The call volume is increasing   131
Discussion   133

Solutions and realignment   134
Takeaways   135
Case 3: System-wide adoption   136
Discussion   139
Solutions and realignment   140
Takeaways   141
Summary   142
References   142

15. Teleneurology in academics   **145**

Jillian Heisler, MD, PhD, Rajan Gadhia, MD

Introduction to virtual care within graduate medical education   145
Final thoughts from trainee and mentee   153
References   153

16. Telehealth laws, regulations, and reimbursement   **155**

George Williams, MD, FASA, FCCM, FCCP, Randall Wright, MD

Introduction   155
Licensure   158
Practice standards   159
Payment   160
References   164
Further reading   164

17. International teleneurology   **165**

Esther Cubo, MD, PhD

Background   165
The burden of neurological disorders   165
Clinical care   166
Other medical specialties   168
Teleneurology toward a preventive medicine and interdisciplinary
    approach   169
Telemedicine programs in underserved areas   170
Humanitarian crisis   172
Education   174
Conclusion   175
References   176

18. Future of telemedicine   **181**
Robert L. Satcher, Jr, MD, PhD

Background/past implementation   181
Current environment   183
Future development and adoption   186
References   191

Index   *195*

Video contents

Chapter 3 The Telestroke evaluation

3.1 NIHSS testing tips

3.2 NIHSS section overview

3.3 Section 1: Level of consciousness

3.4 Section 2: Gaze

3.5 Section 3: Visual field

3.6 Section 4: Facial muscles

3.7 Sections 5-6: Motor exam arms and leg

3.8 Section 7: Ataxia

3.9 Section 8: Sensory

3.10 Section 9: Best language

3.11 Section 10: Dysarthria

3.12 Section 11: Extinction and inattention

Chapter 11 Neuromuscular evaluation

11.1 Virtual examination of facial muscles, facial sensation, and hearing

11.2 Virtual examination of coordination of arms, hands

11.3 Virtual examination of coordination of legs

11.4 Virtual examination of balance and gait

Contributors

Stanley H. Appel, MD
Professor and Chair, Department of Neurology, Houston Methodist Neurological Institute, Houston, TX, United States

Annette E. Brissett, PhD
Director of Psychological Services, Clinical Psychologist, Houston Psychology Consultants; Director of Psychological Services, Clinical Psychologist, Brain Health Consultants and TMS Center, Houston, TX, United States

Gavin W. Britz, MD, MPH, MBA, FAANS
Department of Neurosurgery, Houston Methodist Hospital, Houston, TX, United States

Nhu Bruce, MD
Director of the Houston Methodist Woodlands Stroke Center, Houston, TX, United States

Pablo R. Castillo, MD
Program Director Sleep Fellowship, Neurology, Mayo Clinic, Jacksonville, FL, United States

Esther Cubo, MD, PhD
Neurology Department, Hospital Universitario Burgos, University of Burgos, Burgos, Spain

Garvin Davis, MD, MPH
Director, Retinal Disease and Surgery, The Robert Cizik Eye Clinic, Houston, TX, United States

Rajan Gadhia, MD
Vascular Neurologist, Neurology, Houston Methodist Hospital, Houston, TX, United States

Ronald Goldsberry
Microbiologist, City of Houston, Houston, TX, United States

Ericka Greene, MD
Associate Professor, Education Director of Neurology, Division Head, Neuromuscular Medicine Houston Methodist Neurological Institute; Curriculum Director, Practice of Medicine, EnMed, Texas A&M University College of Medicine, College of Engineering, Houston, TX, United States

Jillian Heisler, MD, PhD
Physician, Neurology, Houston Methodist Hospital, Houston, TX, United States

Paul Holman, MD
Director of Neurosurgical Spine Center and Director of Neurosurgical Spine Fellowship Program, Neurological Surgery; Department of Neurosurgery, Houston Methodist Hospital, Houston, TX, United States

Jonathan J. Lee, MD
Department of Neurosurgery, Houston Methodist Hospital, Houston, TX, United States

Zoltan Mari, MD, FAAN
Ruvo Family Chair, Lou Ruvo Center for Brain Health; Director of Parkinson's & Movement Disorder Program, Lou Ruvo Center for Brain Health, Neurological Institute, Cleveland Clinic; Clinical Professor, Medicine (Neurology), University of Nevada Las Vegas, Las Vegas, NV; Adjunct Associate Professor, Neurology, Johns Hopkins University, Baltimore, MD, United States

Katherine Noe, MD, PhD
Associate Professor of Neurology, Neurology, Mayo Clinic Arizona, Phoenix, AZ, United States

Kenneth Podell, PhD
Director of Houston Methodist Concussion Center, Stanley H Appel Department of Neurology, Houston Methodist; Associate Professor, Clinical Neurology, Weill-Cornell Medical School and Institute of Academic Medicine, Houston, TX, United States

Robert L. Satcher, Jr, MD, PhD
MD Anderson Cancer Center, Houston, TX, United States

Fernando E. Silva, MD
Director of Neurosurgical Spine Center and Director of Neurosurgical Spine Fellowship Program, Neurological Surgery, Houston Methodist Hospital, Houston, TX, United States

Stacy V. Smith, MD
Neuro-Ophthalmologist, Houston Methodist Neurological Institute and Blanton Eye Institute, Woodlands, TX, United States

Stephen Spielman, MBA, MHA
Senior Vice President and Chief Operating Officer, Houston Methodist Physician Organization; President of Primary Care Group, Houston Methodist Hospital, Houston, TX, United States

John J. Volpi, MD
Director of Stroke Division, Houston Methodist Neurological Institute, Houston Methodist Hospital, Houston, TX, United States

George Williams, MD, FASA, FCCM, FCCP
Medical Co-Director, LBJ Surgical Intensive Care Unit; Vice Chair for Critical Care Medicine, UT Houston Department of Anesthesiology, Houston, TX, United States

Randall Wright, MD
Director of the Brain Wellness and Sleep Program, Houston Methodist Hospital, The Woodlands; Clinical Faculty EnMed, Texas A&M University College of Medicine, College of Engineering, Houston, TX, United States

About the editor

Dr. Randall J. Wright is the Director of the Brain Wellness and Sleep Program at Houston Methodist Hospital in the Woodlands, Texas. Dr. Wright also serves as clinical faculty for the EnMed, Texas A&M University College of Medicine, College of Engineering, Houston, TX, United States. Dr. Wright approaches his mission of improving the health of this world from the lenses of science, technology, and creative thinking. He received both a Physics degree from Xavier University of Louisiana and an Electrical Engineering degree from the Georgia Institute of Technology before completing medical school at Emory University and finally Residency and a Clinical Neurophysiology fellowship from Baylor College of Medicine. Beyond his formal education, Dr. Wright developed his executive leadership skills by serving as Chief of Neurology at Conroe Regional Medical Center, Medical Director of the Conroe Regional Neurovascular Stroke Center, Medical Director of the Health South Rehab Stroke Unit, and Assistant Professor of Neurology, Department of Neurosurgery, UT School of Medicine. His community experience ranges from forming the first ever stroke support group in Montgomery County, Texas to working with Washington, DC affiliates of the American Heart Association to shape health policies affecting the nation. Dr. Wright continues to live out his mission to marry technology and science-backed principles of health with real-life implementation in order to dramatically evolve self-care and health care as we know it in order to transform as many lives as possible for the better.

Introduction

The world has changed. Health care has changed. Innovative models of care were needed, and telemedicine has arrived, empowering both patients and physicians. Writing an introduction to these contributions on telemedicine edited by Dr. Randy Wright is truly a privilege. With increasing innovation in technology, our medical world is changing rapidly. Nowhere is this more evident than in the use of telecommunication and information technologies to improve patient services. We have entered an era of "healing from a distance," I share Randy Wright's vision of "telemedicine as the next great contribution to medicine," and this volume is dedicated to educating our neurology colleagues about the opportunities, the challenges, and the promises of applying telemedicine to neurology.

Novel treatments and cures are focused on the future as well as the present. From a practical point of view, telemedicine is the here and now, providing meaningful face-to-face communication between doctors and patients to sustain patients' quality of life given the limitation of in-person visits. Technical innovations have enabled us to reach patients who were previously unreachable. Smartphones are no longer just the province of young adults and children. Older individuals are now becoming increasingly familiar and comfortable communicating with smartphones, and this familiarity can lead the way to improved health care. From a patient's perspective, virtual visits have been enthusiastically welcomed, especially for those living great distances from medical centers. Long car rides take many hours, and the physical hardships of such travel need to be avoided. The unsafe travel from remote distances has been obviated by the virtual visit, and the virtual visit has been necessitated by the onslaught of COVID-19.

The coronavirus pandemic arrived suddenly and unexpectedly, and dramatically changed our approach to medical care. Telemedicine has become an important way to sustain and enhance patients' quality of life. Virtual visits have long provided an opportunity to deliver medical care to patients who live at far distances from tertiary care centers. Yet they were underutilized because it was felt that in-person visits were the only way to provide optimal care. Experience with virtual visits was extremely limited. All this has changed with COVID-19. Patients have been reluctant to travel and even more reluctant to embrace in-person encounters in a hospital setting, fearful of contracting coronavirus if they came to a crowded medical center, especially tertiary medical centers treating a large number of COVID-19 patients. Social distancing also requires avoiding the customary in-person visit, but it does not mandate avoiding medical care.

Delays in seeking medical attention may hamper recognition of evolving neurological deficits which require immediate attention. Patients with chronic neurological diseases have a lowered threshold for other disorders. For example, the patient who has experienced a transient ischemic attack has a risk of further vascular disease, and risks possible coronavirus infection with its ability to impair coagulation and endothelial cell functions. A virtual visit could confirm the patient's status and whether or not hospitalization is required. Patients with many neurodegenerative diseases have comorbidities (such as an Amyotrophic Lateral Sclerosis (ALS) patient with compromised respiratory function) that make them vulnerable to COVID-19. Close monitoring with virtual visits can provide the continuity of care to lessen the impact of comorbidities and minimize the risk of fatal infection.

As the pandemic has lingered, virtual visits have increased dramatically. In early 2020, the priority of our hospitals was caring for COVID-19 cases. Medical facilities were less available to routine follow-up care as well as noncoronavirus new patient visits. In-person visits were extremely limited, and virtual visits were the answer. What was most gratifying was the rapid acceptance of virtual care, even among older adults who had previously only been comfortable with in-person visits. From the perspective of both patients and medical personnel, virtual care was initially the only way to deliver medical care, and is now appreciated and valued as an effective way to deliver quality care. There is less need to postpone medical evaluations or treatments for patients with chronic neurological conditions.

The virtual visits themselves have evolved. They originally represented opportunities limited to taking a history. They have now evolved into more complete evaluations of the patient's medical status, and an opportunity for understanding the 24/7 environment in which the patient is functioning. Missing from in-person visits has been a firsthand look at the home environments and how patients function in that environment. For example, a major concern for our ALS patients is their loss of balance and their frequent falls. They may come into the clinic with walkers and wheelchairs, but they often abandon the use of assistive devices at home. With a look around their home on a virtual visit, a cluttered environment becomes readily apparent, and ways to improve the situation can be suggested. Multiple accidents are just waiting to happen and need to be prevented. Similar insights into problematic situations become apparent with Parkinson's disease patients and aging individuals with cognitive dysfunction; these situations can be addressed, and accidents hopefully avoided.

The chapters in this book address neurological diseases, where virtual visits can provide in-depth evaluations. What is mandated is that the medical team develop the know-how and the skills to elicit information during virtual visits that is somewhat comparable to what has been so effectively practiced over many years of in-person examinations. We readily recognize that virtual visits cannot easily substitute for the warmth and emotional support of the in-person visit. Doctors customarily approach in-patient visits with a desire to comfort and problem-solve; patients similarly have confidence that they will benefit from the visit with the doctor. There is real value in the unspoken emotional connection and the implied contract. The virtual visit needs to recognize the therapeutic importance of establishing a strong bond of confidence between doctor and patient. Empathy is the hallmark of the successful visit, whether in-person or at home.

Nevertheless, the challenges can be daunting. To carry out a successful virtual visit, not only is emotional support required, but so is the patient and family's technological expertise, and this may be limited by the patient's lack of knowledge and/or finances. The widespread availability of smartphones makes this issue less of a concern, except for the truly impoverished—those same individuals whose access to in-person visits is extremely constricted. An additional challenge is that patients with chronic neurological diseases may not be capable of effective communication, and the success of the visit depends very much on family support. Thus, both patient and family members need to be educated as to what is required for the most beneficial outcome. Family members especially need to be committed and involved in their loved one's care.

The next generation of virtual visits should provide a quantum leap in information available remotely. Neurological functions are being increasingly monitored with techniques that have been validated in the clinic and now can be administered at home, and downloaded for continuous assessment. In ALS, for example, changes in speech can be readily quantitated with smartphone evaluations. Respiratory function can also be monitored with a spirometer connected to a smartphone. Muscle strength is evaluated with a handheld dynamometer. Overall function is readily assessed with the ALS Functional Rating Scale, which has long been validated from in-person visits and can be readily administered either over the phone or at home by the patient and family. All of these tools provide a meaningful evaluation of the status of the patient, and when carried out on an ongoing basis, we can determine not only the burden of disease, but rates of disease progression as well. In the chapters that follow, novel tools and techniques of home evaluations are presented that can similarly evaluate the burden of disease and rates of progression in different neurological conditions; their validation and utilization will dramatically enhance the value of virtual visits.

The past lack of reimbursement definitely limited widespread adoption of telemedicine, despite evidence that remote care by a neurologist yielded outcomes comparable to in-patient visits. During the pandemic, telemedicine visits have increased dramatically, fueled primarily by the increased need, but as well in large part by the Centers of Medicare & Medicaid Services (CMS) and commercial payers reimbursing care. Acceptance by both patients and medical professionals has been so great that if the financial barriers can be lifted and reimbursement continued on an ongoing basis, as much as 30% of ongoing follow-up care might be virtual. We cannot lose what has been a tremendous advance in medical care. Telemedicine has been phenomenally successful in meeting medical and patient needs, and government and private insurers should be urged to continue to reimburse these beneficial home evaluations as a major milestone in leading medicine and improving the quality of life for our patients.

Stanley H. Appel, MD
Professor and Chair, Department of Neurology, Houston Methodist
Neurological Institute, Houston, TX, United States

CHAPTER 1

Responding to a crisis: A call to action

Stephen Spielman, MBA, MHA[a,b]
[a]Senior Vice President and Chief Operating Officer, Houston Methodist Physician Organization, Houston Methodist Hospital, Houston, TX, United States
[b]President of Primary Care Group, Houston Methodist Hospital, Houston, TX, United States

Introduction

As coronavirus disease 2019 (COVID-19) escalated into a global pandemic, health system scrambled to prepare for surge conditions. Patient loads increased exponentially, and state governmental agencies advised hospitals to double their capacity while simultaneously reducing their non–COVID-19 patient populations. As an additional measure to free up bed capacity, nonemergent medical procedures were severely restricted. The pressure to prepare and the pressure to perform changed how health care was delivered during that time and, potentially, permanently.

I am the Senior Vice President of the Houston Methodist Physician Organization, which employs 800 physicians across 18 specialties in 170 clinics across a geography larger than the state of Connecticut. Our Houston Methodist Hospital system includes eight hospitals, an integrated academic institute, and Houston Methodist (HM) operates more than 2393 hospital beds and has approximately 25,000 employees. Some changes at Houston Methodist were consistent with preparations modeled around the world, but others offer case studies for the future. With the dedicated and coordinated efforts of our hospital employees, our academic and clinical staff, our government leaders, and our first responders, this pandemic will end. However, the effects on hospitals and how we deliver care in physician offices may forever be changed. In many ways, health care will never be the same—and that is a very good thing.

Virtual foundation

In the months leading up to COVID-19, Houston Methodist was celebrating a milestone of success as we had reached a pace of 1000 visits per month through our "on demand" virtual urgent care platform. HM physicians and

1

advanced practice nurses were employed to be "at the ready" to treat specific common medical conditions through a mobile virtual interface. Our virtual urgent care platform was accessible in a number of online venues such as Walgreens and Zocdoc. We had seen a volume increase of 20% every month in patient visits, had outstanding patient satisfaction scores, and the platform was proving to offer a cost-effective way to treat common illness in the comfort of the patient's own home. The data we collected from those seeking virtual urgent care showed that many individuals were using this form of care delivery to supplant primary care office visits or urgent care visit (Fig. 1.1).

In our established physician practices, we were utilizing our EMR, EPIC, to deliver virtual care to our patients that needed specialty and primary care. Patient volume was low in this use case, as we were struggling to implement a new virtual care operational workflow in a traditional practice. There was not a "burning bridge" moment to spur our physicians to try virtual care. We found that often times, physicians would be very excited about the idea of virtual care and would want to pilot it in their clinics. However, when it came time to introduce the new workflow, the momentum of the traditional in-person style of visits would quickly suffocate any new process. In the end, adoption for virtual care in established physician practices was low. It was clear that although we had made tremendous strides in building the

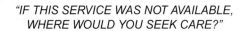

"IF THIS SERVICE WAS NOT AVAILABLE, WHERE WOULD YOU SEEK CARE?"

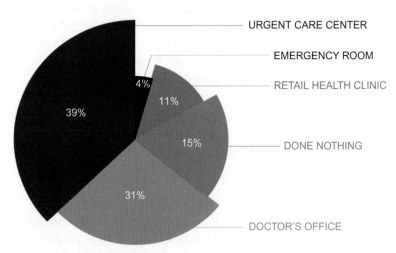

Fig. 1.1 Virtual care patient preference survey results.

administrative and IT infrastructure to facilitate a virtual health platform, many physicians were skeptical or felt like the time for virtual care had not come—at least not yet.

It was clear that we were at the beginning of a very long journey. We had a clear strategic imperative to build new patient business, reduce facility overhead, be more consumer-centric, and maintain connectivity with our patient base by leveraging virtual medical care. In our most optimistic of moments, we would hope that we could get 50% physician adoption of virtual care in our established physician offices, and reach 2000 patient visits per month on our virtual urgent care platform in the next 3 years. We had no idea of the impending wave of adoption that would push our dreams of virtual care to the brink and serve as a foundation of stability that we would use as a base for our slow and steady recovery from the worst pandemic in 100 years.

COVID-19

Being located close to the Gulf of Mexico, Houston Methodist (HM) is used to dealing with significant weather events, such as hurricanes and tropical storms. We are used to dealing with disasters and their associated recoveries. We know how to set up incident command infrastructures and deliver care to our patients in time of significant need. Five years ago, HM navigated through hurricane Harvey, a 100-year hurricane that resulted in historic flooding of the Houston area. We learned significantly from these types of events about how to deal with natural disasters. These organizational skills of resiliency, necessary organizational infrastructure, along with our complete dedication to our core values of integrity, compassion, accountability, and excellence to help guide our decision-making would serve us well in the fight that was to come against COVID-19.

At the beginning of March 2020, COVID-19 was starting to impact operational decisions significantly in the Houston Methodist Physician Organization, and how we deliver care to our patients. We immediately fell into a similar routine, as if battling a hurricane. We opened our "incident command infrastructure" and proceeded to prioritize our efforts. We immediately took stock of our assets to come up with a compressive plan to see patients in a safe outpatient (OP) clinical environment. At that time, we were unsure how COVID-19 was transmitted, how to disinfect our clinics properly between patients, or what assurances we could give our staff that they could work in a safe environment. Operating clinical operations with this amount of uncertainty left us with little choice but to switch most scheduled OP clinic visits to virtual visits. This would require an incredible effort by our physicians, operational teams, and all support services. Within our organization, we see on average 40,000 visits per month and employ more than 800 physicians over 15 clinical specialties. To transition our traditional in-person clinical care model successfully to a virtual care delivery model, the following would have to be accomplished:

1. **Training**—all physicians and staff would have to be trained on the in-place EPIC EMR technology that would facilitate virtual care.
2. **Patient education**—patients would have to be notified of this change in their appointments. Support lines would need to be established to help patients through technological difficulties. Physicians and staff would need talking points to ease patients' fears/concerns about being treated virtually.
3. **Technology enhancement**—we would need additional software server space so our technology could work efficiently. In-place technology to facilitate virtual care was not scaled to accommodate the volumes we were preparing to deliver.
4. **Communication**—the organization needed to be in-sync to deliver a consistent message regarding our switch to virtual care, so that we could maintain the confidence of the community that we served.

Training

The lessons learned in our pre-COVID-19 virtual care experiences became invaluable for us to spring into action. Prior to COVID-19, we only had a small population of physicians who were willing to accept, or even try, a virtual approach to care delivery. Common excuses given were: "No way you can effectively treat someone virtually," "My patients don't want this," or "This is not how I was trained." These responses to virtual care quickly subsided when left with an option of not treating patients or finding a way to make virtual care work for their patient population. We immediately seized on the change in momentum and within 24 h we were setting up webinars, in-person training presentations, and printing "tip sheets" explaining how to perform a virtual outpatient clinic visit. The reception from the physician community to the training and move to virtual was incredibly positive. Physicians were excited that we had found a way to treat their patients safely and were relieved that the virtual visit platform was intuitive and easy to learn. Everyone understood that this was a new process and there were

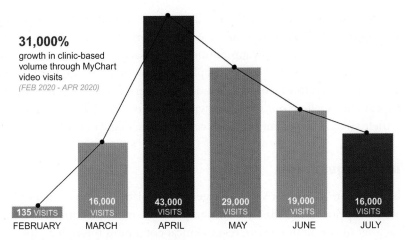

Fig. 1.2 Growth in virtual care trended by month.

inherent glitches in the system that would have to be worked out. Within 3 weeks, we had effectively converted 80% of our visits to a virtual setting, and we trained 900 physicians in under 2 weeks (Fig. 1.2).

The organization was coming together to find a way for our patients to be treated, and at an amazing implementation speed. It was a time of crisis, which galvanized us to make use of this new platform that we always knew had potential.

Communication

The pandemic was fully upon us and the related information concerning how one might be infected was changing daily as the science community was further understanding the disease. As fast as we were coming together to fight this virus as an institution, we understood we had to educate and support our patients quickly in this time of uncertainty. We had to deliver a message to our patient panels that we were here to support them through all things COVID-19, as well as to treat them for non-COVID-19 related illnesses. Our patients were scared and needed reassuring. We immediately started a city-wide marketing campaign to educate them not only on our virtual platform, but also that we were there for them in their time of need. Communication on a mass scale was necessary, but we also wanted to convey a more personal message to each patient. Two years prior to COVID-19, we invested in a bi-directional, Health Insurance Portability and Accountability Act (HIPPA)-compliant, text-based communication platform that allows us to text our patients directly and allows them to text us back with any concerns they have. We commonly use this platform to deliver appointment reminders, or any other preappointment necessary information. Our patients became comfortable using this platform to communicate with us. We immediately used this technology to deliver a personalized text message to each patient, detailing our move to a virtual platform to deliver patient care for their safety. The patient response was overwhelmingly positive.

Virtual urgent care

The Houston Methodist Virtual Urgent Care platform had been in place for 2 years prior to COVID-19. On this platform, nurse practitioners would treat a set of common nonemergent clinical conditions through a Houston Methodist Hospital mobile application via a synchronous live person visit. The experience was very similar to Facetime on the Apple IOS system. Throughout COVID-19, this delivery system has seen record numbers of visits from patients who were fearful of COVID-19 exposure, had contracted COVID-19, or wanted reassurance about how this disease is spreading. Within the first few days of the pandemic event, we were immediately overwhelmed with patient appointments. The third-party, virtual care IT platform we were utilizing to perform these visits was struggling to maintain server infrastructure to keep up with demand. The platform was experiencing IT issues nationally, which was affecting our ability to perform these visits efficiently. We also struggled with finding enough providers to put on the platform to meet the huge demand. Within a few weeks, we regained our operational stability and were able to meet the demand coming our way. This was accomplished by our primary care doctors volunteering to conduct virtual visits, and by hard work by both our internal operations and IT teams. The virtual urgent care program had grown exponentially in only a few months (Fig. 1.3).

Patient feedback

While we were amazed at the growth, the question remained: "Do our patients like our virtual care platform?" To answer this question, we sent out patient satisfaction surveys to those who had completed a virtual visit with Houston Methodist in an effort to garner feedback and refine our platform. The returned surveys were incredibly promising. During the pandemic, our Press Ganey patient satisfaction scores reached over the 90th percentile.

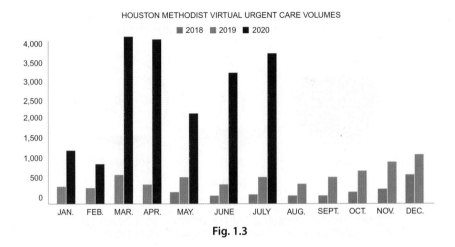

Fig. 1.3

Patients were incredibly thankful that we were able to maintain connectivity to them throughout this time and address their COVID-19 concerns, as well as treat their non-COVID-19 chronic conditions. It was clear these new virtual platforms were not only useful, but also enjoyed by our patients due to the convenience and safety offered.

Physician feedback

Even as we were fighting COVID-19, we were planning for what "virtual care" would look like in the future. The first step in our planning process was to get feedback from our physicians, who were collectively seeing more than 3000 patients every day on the virtual platform. We asked questions related to transition, ease of use, clinical efficacy, and future adoption. The results of each question were very insightful. We were pleased to see the high marks related to overall transition to the virtual platform from a traditional in-person setting (Fig. 1.4).

The feedback was used to create an "onboarding tool set" for our new physicians, who were interested in learning how to perform virtual medicine in their clinics. Physicians were also very interested in continuing to see both new and established patients in their clinic virtually after the COVID-19 pandemic subsides (Fig. 1.5).

Many physicians noted that the ease of use, the increase in efficiency, and patient satisfaction were key drivers in making this decision. Given the feedback, we assembled a small group of physician leaders interested in pursuing future capabilities in outpatient virtual health. This group offered

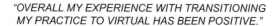

"OVERALL MY EXPERIENCE WITH TRANSITIONING MY PRACTICE TO VIRTUAL HAS BEEN POSITIVE."

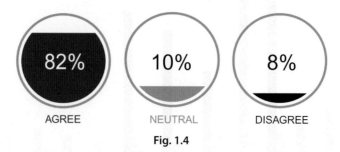

Fig. 1.4

"ONCE THINGS NORMALIZE AFTER COVID, I WOULD LIKE TO CONTINUE USING VIRTUAL VISITS IN MY PRACTICE."

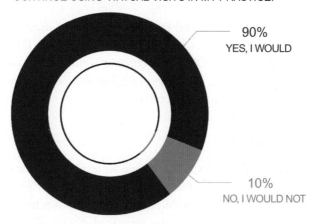

Fig. 1.5

ideas on future virtual connectivity between primary care and specialty care physicians to treat patients in a single outpatient office visit. Above all, we wanted to ensure that clinical decision-making and appropriate referral making could be maintained while on a virtual platform. The results indicated (Fig. 1.6) that for the most part, virtual health did not hinder a physician's ability to evaluate a patient.

However, when it came to the ability to make an appropriate referral, the responses were mixed (Fig. 1.7).

Thirty-five percent of the physicians surveyed felt that they were not able to refer patients to the appropriate physicians for specialty care to the same degree, when compared to evaluating a patient in-person. Physicians noted two major obstacles to the referral workflow: (1) the outpatient clinic

DO PHYSICIANS FEEL THEY ARE ABLE TO GET ENOUGH
CLINICAL INFORMATION DURING VIRTUAL VISITS?

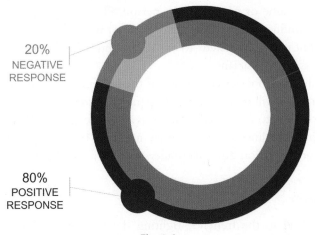

20%
NEGATIVE
RESPONSE

80%
POSITIVE
RESPONSE

Fig. 1.6

"WHEN YOU CONSIDER REFERRING A PATIENT TO
A SPECIALIST, ARE YOU ABLE TO DO THIS TO THE
SAME DEGREE AS WHEN YOU SEE THEM IN CLINIC?"

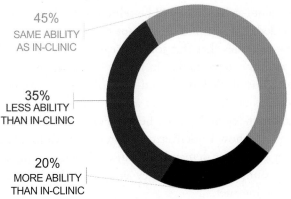

45%
SAME ABILITY
AS IN-CLINIC

35%
LESS ABILITY
THAN IN-CLINIC

20%
MORE ABILITY
THAN IN-CLINIC

Fig. 1.7

support staff not being in place to facilitate a smooth virtual referral; and
(2) patients needed to be further educated on the virtual platform technology to complete the visits. These two findings highlighted a need for us to
reengineer our outpatient clinical workflow to better facilitate virtual visits
for our patients. We needed to make sure physicians had dedicated time to
complete the virtual visits and medical assistants needed to be trained on

how to coach the patient to be seen virtually. The remaining 65% of physicians surveyed felt that they were able to refer to the appropriate specialist about the same or more than in-person. These were encouraging data, giving us confidence that our legacy referral process did not need to be "rebuilt" but rather "tweaked" to ensure an optimal referral experience for our patients and physicians.

Virtual care is not perfect. We are at the beginning of long journey that we must realize will have significant operational challenges. It is imperative that we continue to listen to the opinions and experiences of physicians and staff on the front lines so that we may improve. To that end, we continue to survey and question our stakeholders regularly on what we can improve.

Conclusion

As we are still in the trenches, fighting the COVID-19 pandemic with every resource that we have, planning for a COVID-19-free future may seem unrealistic or burdensome. However, organizations must evaluate what new processes are working now so that they may be expanded upon in the future. How patients receive care may be forever changed due to this pandemic. Medicare and other large national payers have signaled that payment for virtual patient care services will be reimbursed—however, at what level is still undecided. This seismic movement by the payers to pay for virtual health all but solidifies that this form of care is here to stay. To that end, virtual care is now a new market in health care and there are new players such as Apple, Amwell, Walgreens, and Amazon, which have taken notice of the opportunities to disintermediate a very clunky health care system by offering consumer-focused virtual health. For health systems to compete, we must also learn how to deliver care faster, more easily, and more effectively to meet consumer demand. We must get better at delivering virtual health to meet our patients where they already conduct a large part of their transactions: the internet.

CHAPTER 2

The telemedicine exam general overview

Randall Wright, MD^{a,b}, Ronald Goldsberry^c
^aDirector of the Brain Wellness and Sleep Program, Houston Methodist Hospital, The Woodlands, TX, United States
^bClinical Faculty EnMed, Texas A&M University College of Medicine, College of Engineering, Houston, TX, United States
^cMicrobiologist, City of Houston, Houston, TX, United States

The concept of telemedicine has been part of our human experience since ancient history, and really parallels the advancement in communication over the centuries. The idea of being able to communicate medical information over a long distance has been necessary since the onset of the healing arts. The need to communicate birth or death notices, details of a plague outbreak, or the extent of battle injuries have been challenging doctors and inventors over the ages. Early versions of long-distance communication of medical information have been reported to include modalities such as smoke signals, drums, and even flag semaphores (those oddly marked flags people often wave on military vessels). The invention of the telegraph propelled civilization into a new age of electronic communication and arguably initiated the early renditions of modern telemedicine. The telegraph soon became the telephone and the use of the more reliable means of long-distance communication became immensely popular, especially in the military. Doctors and military personnel could now order supplies, communicate injury and casualty counts, and even perform doctor-to-doctor consultations over long distances.

A long list of pioneers forged the way for the development of telemedicine. Willem Einthoven, inventor of the electrocardiograph, started developing the idea of the use of the telephone for remote consultations in 1906. One of the first publicized modern ideas of "telemedicine" appeared in Hugo Gernsback's April 1924 issue of *Radio News Magazine*. Despite the periodical being a radio-based magazine, it took a very advanced look into what health care could be if we used a television equipped with a microphone to facilitate communication between doctors and patients.

Traditionally, the first real-time audio-video telemedicine consult is often credited to the University of Nebraska in 1959 when doctors performed a neurological exam on a psychiatric patient. From there an interactive network between Logan International Airport and Massachusetts General Hospital in the 1960s developed into a true telemedicine network.

Telemedicine has been a dream in the minds of innovators for many years. As we just reviewed, there have been many trailblazers who have worked tirelessly to give us a vision of the future and how health care could evolve to serve an even greater good. As with all visionary ideas, after the honeymoon of thought is over, the reality of implementation sets in and a whole host of deterrents begin to emerge. The practical and widespread adaptation of telemedicine has been slowed over recent years due to appropriate concerns of privacy, regulation, ability, and acceptance. HIPPA has outlined clear guidelines for addressing privacy concerns for visits conducted via telemedicine means. Government regulation and health insurance reimbursement practices are an evolving topic, have but becoming more favorable as time passes. Acceptance was the "bogeyman" that often hid in the back of the minds of individuals who were new to telemedicine and were skeptical of their patient's acceptance a virtual visit over a live-in-person visit. Well, the COVID-19 pandemic has basically revealed that such concerns, though valid, may be less of a barrier that we initially thought. In March of 2020, we as medical professions were faced with a "burning building" scenario of either closing down our offices due to governmental shutdown orders or finding other ways to care for our patients' needs. In this "stay and burn" or "jump" scenario, many of us chose to jump. In this case, the leap of faith was to jump into this questionable space of telemedicine. Providers across the world seemingly overnight temporarily closed the doors to their traditional office-based practice of medicine and entered the virtual world of jacket, blouse/shirt and tie, sweatpants, and the onset of the virtual visit! Practitioners were not alone in this leap of faith. Local medical boards, governors, President Donald Trump, and insurance companies alike, to our surprise, immediately removed nearly all of the regulatory barriers to telehealth, and our ability to care for patients transitioned into the 21st century. We were all suddenly ushered into caring for a variety of medical conditions that we, just the week before, had thought could only be handled in person (because that is all we knew how to do). Doctors and patients were finally sitting in the classroom of life together and learned how to relate medically to one another in a virtual space. As the weeks went on, we learned that patients actually enjoyed the convenience of seeing their doctor from the comfort of their own home. Doctors realized the efficiency and convenience of virtual visits and that topics that were once thought impossible (i.e., the medical exam) were actually possible.

This book serves as a punctuation point in the history of telemedicine, specifically in the neurosciences. The voices you will hear in the book come from around the world and wish to articulate where we are "today" and to nod to where we may be in the future. This book and the following chapters are designed to express to you the reality of this changing component of the practice of medicine. We by no means intend to state that telemedicine is a defined field that has all the answers. By contrast, we acknowledge that clear guidelines, research, and data in the virtual practice of medicine re limited and ongoing. We acknowledge that many chapters and concepts are being articulated for the first time and may be imperfect. To that end, the authors involved in this project have agreed to revisit these topics 4–5 years from now and update you on any progress. So, with this background being laid, let's turn the proverbial page on the in-person neurological evaluation and let's start to understand the components of the virtual neurological evaluation of a patient.

The virtual visit

When preparing for your televisit, it is good to start with the end in mind. There has been a lot of experience with telemedicine now, and we are starting to see a few trends in the research about what makes a televisit successful. There is a growing number of research papers about patient perceptions of virtual visits and lessons learned from such interactions. One such article published by the Mayo Clinic[1] recounts feedback from 49,000 patient comments over an 11-month period. Their overall findings suggested that the patients who were most satisfied with their visit appreciated the relationship that they established with their provider. The Mayo Clinic argued that the key elements to establishing a good virtual patient-doctor relationship from the perspective of patients was mainly focused on the communication skill of the provider and was less focused on the patient's receipt of a prescription. The study supported the notion that a patient-doctor relationship can effectively be established through a video consultation when the provider focuses on patient-centered relationship building. This brings us back to the basic tenet of health care. The base word is "care" and that should be your focus. The ability to exhibit empathy, compassion, and attentiveness has been found to be a key element that makes a great doctor and will help you have a great virtual visit with your patients.

The key premise in setting yourself up for a successful virtual visit in the eyes of your patient is to start the visit with the right mindset. Yes, our goal is to make an accurate assessment of the patient's medical concerns, decide on the need for appropriate diagnostic testing, make a diagnosis, and then prescribe appropriate treatment. That is the basic requirement of being a physician and the basic assumption of what your patient expects from you. That is equivalent to going to a fast food restaurant, ordering a hamburger, and receiving a burger, bun, tomato slice, and shred of lettuce. Yes, you have received a hamburger and that thing you received will fulfill your basic request for sustenance and possibly taste, but will you enjoy it? Probably not, when compared to another restaurant that uses toasted buns with sesame seeds, flame-broiled organic buffalo meat patties with a special rub seasoning, freshly harvested tomatoes, lettuce, pickles, and onions from a locally grown garden topped off with an in-house-made sauce. It's as if this burger was made with you in mind, and I bet you will love it more! Both are burgers, both have the necessary components of providing you with a meal, but the one that you most enjoy has all the extras made just for you. It is the same with your televisit. When you approach your visit with the mindset of getting to know your patient, providing them with a structure for the virtual visit, listening to their story, and providing them with appropriate education and guidance, your efforts are more likely to be received in a much more positive light.

The basics of communication skills needed to perform an in-person medical examination have been taught in medical school for years. In 2001, the essential elements of physician–patient communication were examined in depth to provide guidance for medical schools and standards for professional practice. The culmination of such research was discussed in a 3-day conference in Kalamazoo, Michigan in May of 1999. The proceedings became known as the Kalamazoo Consensus Statement and were published by Gregory Makoul. This group identified seven essential elements of a good doctor-patient relationship, and these are outlined in Table 2.1.

Table 2.1 The seven essential sets of communication tasks by the Kalamazoo consensus.[2]

1. Build the doctor-patient relationship
2. Open the discussion
3. Gather information
4. Understand the patient's perspective
5. Share information
6. Reach agreement on problems and plans
7. Provide closure

These key elements have been echoed across every first-year medical school to some degree and are timeless treasures. However, in our busy everyday practice where the demands to see more patients becomes ever more daunting, these rapport building techniques may often be sacrificed for more direct means, or a patriarchal doctor–patient relationship. When entering the virtual age of health care, it becomes more and more important to practice a more patient-centered style of practice. Studies have shown that physicians who are skilled in conveying emotion through both verbal and nonverbal means of communications are perceived in a more positive light by their patients, as evidenced through patient satisfaction scores.[3–5] The importance of the use of nonverbal communication skills to improve the physician–patient relationship is being recognized more now as an essential part of health care and being emphasized more in medical training programs around the world. This skill set is even more critical in the virtual world. The ability to convey emotion, empathy and develop an authentic connection with your patient in the virtual world will be a necessary skill to ensure your success in the practice of telemedicine. To go into detail of how to demonstrate empathy and emotion to your patients is beyond the scope of this book, but it is worth noting that you do have certain tools in your toolbox to help you convey to your patients the emotional message required. Many of the tools you will use to express emotion will be nonverbal.[6,7] Many authors have written on the variety of ways in which nonverbal communication can convey significant messages to your patients.[5,8–10] Table 2.2 lists some of the tools you have to assist you in conveying nonverbal messages to your patients effectively.

In the virtual world, these tools and the attempt to forge emotional connections with your patient can be summed up in the popular new term "webside manner."[11] The term represents that translation of old-fashioned bedside manner into its virtual equivalent. The rules for establishing rapport

Table 2.2 Nonverbal behaviors involved in expressing emotion.

1. Facial expressivity (smiling, frowning, etc.)
2. Eye contact (want to make more)
3. Paralinguistic speech characteristics such as rate of speech, pitch, loudness of voice, and pauses
4. Head nodding (to show agreement)
5. Hand gestures (to help demonstrate or add emphasis)
6. Postural positions (open or closed body posture and forward to backward body lean)

have been described above. However, for your virtual visit, we are not quite done yet. There are a few more technical considerations that you need to review, and the next section will walk you through it.

Technical aspects of the virtual visit

Lights, camera, action! These may not be the typical concepts we as physicians think about, but interestingly enough, if you are to be successful in the telehealth world, you will need to be familiar with such concepts, but on a smaller scale. When it comes to performing a virtual visit, it is important to set your stage for a successful encounter. The technology devices you use will affect how your visit is perceived by your patients.

Many authors on this topic suggest having a checklist of important elements of your video visit.[1, 11] Such a list is helpful as you get started, but over time it should become more natural. So, let's start with the basic setup of your virtual visit environment. Have a high-definition camera located at eye level. Make sure this camera has a high-quality built-in microphone, or have an external microphone that is placed out of view of the camera. Whether you are performing virtual visits at the office or at home, you need to designate a special space from which to perform your visit. Make sure the space is quiet and private (you don't want other office workers or even children walking into the background of your video visit). Ensure you have a reliable high-speed internet connection. Placing a light source in front of you will highlight your face and minimize shadows. It is helpful to test your lighting before your actual first video visit, to make sure there are no glares or overexposure from the light. Try to avoid having an open window behind you, for too much light behind you may turn you into a dark shadow to the patient. The decor of the background should be simple and nondistracting. Using solid colors can help to enhance the patient's experience by allowing you to be the center of attention. Having too many personal items or books in the background may draw attention away from you. Displaying your medical degree is acceptable in many institutions and should be done where possible. Make sure you sit in the center of the camera view. You should dress in the same clothes that you would wear at your clinic. And most importantly, smile and greet your patients with a warm and friendly introduction.

When preparing for your virtual clinic, it is important to review the timing of the visits in advance. Will your appointments be 15 min, 30 min, or even longer? Working this out will allow you to calculate how much time you have to accomplish your goals during the visit. In addition to reviewing your schedule, I have found it helpful to have quick access to your patient's phone number, in the event that you get disconnected or the audio part of the video visit does not work. And if you do have technical difficulties, the best thing to do is to relax. Many people are doing video visits now, and life happens. Since the COVID-19 pandemic began, we have been in a new work-from-home world. Everyone is using up bandwidth during peak hours for performing telemedicine visits, conference calls, and home schooling. You may have set up the fastest connection possible, but still have problems with the connection (remember, the patient needs good Wi-Fi or cellular service as well). If your patient is in a rural area, problems may occur despite your best efforts. If connection problems occur, having the patient's phone number handy is a good way to save the visit and keep the process moving. Many providers have a video visit prep introduction sheet for their patients, or have their staff orient the patient with the software required. That is a good time to ask the patient to have a backup phone line available for the doctor to call if the video visit is interrupted. Having this backup plan articulated to the patient in advance and having the preferred phone number readily available can reduce anxiety and frustration if technical difficulties are encountered during the video visit.

Once you are on the video call, remember to look directly into the camera and not to stare at your patient's face on the screen. Looking directly into the camera during the visit will give the perception that you are looking directly at the patient, and this is important for building rapport. This takes practice, for we all naturally want to look at the patient's eyes on the screen. Taking notes during the video visit is often another challenge. Many physicians use electronic medical records (EMRs) that have to share the same screen as the video visit program. Thus, physicians are trying to look at the patient and take notes in the EMRs at the same time. This may be perceived by the patient as the physician not paying attention. Some ways to solve this issue include writing your notes after the visit and jotting down information on paper while listening to the patient. Alternatively, you can inform the patient at the start of the visit that you will be taking notes and that they may hear you typing or see you glancing away, but you will be listening and it is OK for them to continue to speak. Having the ability to "read the room" by having a sense of when the patient is conveying to you more emotional information than medical details would be a great time to stop typing, lean in, look directly into the camera, and give the patient reassuring nods. When you are asking more medical timeline-style questions, this may be a good time to type. You will develop your own style over time, but I personally find that patients are very understanding, especially if you communicate to them clearly what is going on and convey your sincere interest in them through both verbal and nonverbal means during the visit.

Body language is often referenced in the literature as an important aspect of nonverbal communication. When performing a video visit, you should be aware that body language can be a powerful tool to enhance your patient's experience. Nods of understanding help the patient to know that you are listening. Leaning forward suggests interest while crossing your arms or leaning back indicates the opposite. Sitting up straight and occasionally leaning forward can convey volumes to your patient. You can also walk the fine line of using appropriate hand movements. Too many hand movements can be distracting, but well-timed gestures can be a great asset to your video visit. Be aware of any nervous habits you may have and avoid tapping, clicking, or fidgeting with objects around you. Some microphones are very sensitive and that tiny sound of your tapping pen may be amplified and distracting to your patient.

Now that you have all the previsit setup completed, and you understand the importance of eye contact and body language, it is time to start speaking to the patient. Of course, the first thing you do is introduce yourself. After the pleasantries, you should verify that they can see and hear you clearly. If you have a backup number to call, inform the patient that if you get disconnected for any reason and cannot rejoin the video call, you will call them on the designated number to decide on the next steps. Once you have set the expectations for the video visit, you can start your consultation. The type of history you take and level of physical exam you perform will depend on the conditions you are evaluating. For specific types of neurological conditions, please see later chapters for helpful tips. At the end of the video visit, you will need to give specific instructions for follow-up. It is helpful in virtual visit appointments to review your treatment plan and give the patient time to ask any questions. When the call is done, it is helpful to allow the patient to hang up first. This avoids the scenario where the patient has one last question but you hung up before they could ask. Such a situation could lead to a cumbersome attempt by the patient to reconnect with you or to call your office to relay a message to you. So, the best way to avoid this inconvenience is to let the patient hang up first, thus ensuring all their questions have been answered, and it also makes you seem patient.

Video visit checklist

Scheduling the visit	1. Have your staff give instruction on how to use the video software or how to download the app.
	2. Have your staff get a contact number for you to call if the video visit gets interrupted.
Before the visit	1. Make sure your video office space is neatly decorated, preferably with solid colors for decor.
	2. Select a quiet location with low probability of interruptions.
	3. Check that the HD camera and microphone(s) are working/turned on.
	4. Ensure that the light source is in front of the camera pointing toward you, and no light sources are behind you (e.g., open windows).
	5. Make sure the Wi-Fi connection is stable.
	6. Ensure you are dressed professionally.
During a video visit	1. Look into the camera to ensure proper eye contact.
	2. Introduce yourself and verify the patient can see and hear you properly.
	3. Inform the patient that if you get disconnected, they should not worry; you will call their provided phone number for further instructions.
	4. Use positive body language to build rapport (nodding, leaning forward, using appropriate hand gestures).
	5. Listen to the patient intently.
	6. Document in a nondistracting manner.
	7. Do not eat or drink during the call.
	8. Avoid using lots of abbreviations or jargon and keep concepts simple, so the patient can really understand what you are thinking and trying to express.
	9. At the end of the visit, restate the plan, give instructions for follow-up if needed, and let the patient hang up first.

These tips on how to prepare for and perform a general video visit are only the beginning of your virtual experience. Granted, the history is a major part of your patient assessment, but there is clearly more. The neurological exam, as we learned earlier, was really the incident case for all other telemedicine evaluations. Thus, as admirers of the neurological sciences, it is now time to dive deeper into the neurological assessment via telemedicine. In the chapters that follow, you will learn how to evaluate a patient with various disorders of the nervous system. You will learn tips on history taking and techniques on the virtual neurological examination. Good luck in your journey.

References

1. Elliot T, Tong I, Sherdan A. Beyond convenience: patients' perceptions of physician interactional skills and compassion via telemedicine. *Mayo Clin Proc.* 2020;4(3):305–314.
2. Makoul G. Essential elements of communication in medical encounters: the Kalamazoo consensus statement. *Acad Med.* 2001;76(4):390–393.
3. DiMatteo MR, Taranta A, Friedman HS, Prince LM. Predicting patient satisfaction from physicians' nonverbal communication skills. *Med Care.* 1980;18:376–387.
4. Friedman HS, DiMatteo MR, Taranta A. A study of the relationship between individual differences in nonverbal expressiveness and factors in personality and social interaction. *J Res Pers.* 1980;14:351–364.
5. DiMatteo MR, Hays RD, Prince LM. Relationship of physicians' nonverbal communication skill to patient satisfaction, appointment noncompliance, and physician workload. *Health Psychol.* 1986;5:581–594.
6. Roter DL, Frankel RM, Hall JA, Sluyter D. The expression of emotion through nonverbal behavior in medical visits: mechanisms and outcomes. *J Gen Intern Med.* 2006;21(Suppl 1):S28–S34.
7. Knapp ML, Hall JA. *Nonverbal Communication in Human Interaction.* 6th ed. Belmont, CA: Wadsworth; 2005.
8. Heath C. *Body Movement and Speech in Medical Interaction.* Cambridge, UK: Cambridge University Press; 1986.
9. Hall JA, Harrigan JA, Rosenthal R. Nonverbal behavior in clinician-patient interaction. *Appl Prev Psychol.* 1995;4:21–37.
10. Oatley K, Jenkins JM. *Understanding Emotions.* Cambridge, MA: Blackwell; 1996.
11. Khosla S. Implementation of synchronous telemedicine into clinical practice. *Sleep Med Clin.* 2020;14(3):347–358.

CHAPTER 3

The TeleStroke evaluation

Nhu Bruce, MD

Director of the Houston Methodist Woodlands Stroke Center, Houston, TX, United States

With the early studies of cerebral perfusion during cerebral ischemia, it is widely known that the rapid restoration of blood flow greatly impacts the extent of infarct related neuronal damage and limits potential stroke sequelae. The thrombolytic trials of the 1990s have cemented the role of IV tPA in acute stroke management, but even with the existence of effective treatment, there were still only a minority of eligible patients receiving the medications. One of the barriers to care was access to a stroke-trained physician capable of assessing and identifying patients eligible for acute intervention. Early on, researchers and clinicians in the field of stroke hypothesized that there was a role for telemedicine in overcoming those limitations to access, and studies have shown that patients who are evaluated by a stroke specialist are more likely to be diagnosed with cerebral ischemia and receive acute interventions such as thrombolytic therapy.

The NIH Stroke Scale (NIHSS) is the tool that has been most widely used by clinicians and researchers to assess the severity of stroke symptoms. It has been repeatedly validated with proven interrater reliability. A study published by Lyden et al. in 1994 demonstrated that study investigators can be certified to use the NIHSS through video training with good and reliable consensus. This video has gone on to be utilized by most research, academic, and hospital institutions to train and certify medical and research staff; annual recertification is generally required. Additionally, the scale also allows for quick and reliable evaluation during a video telemedicine assessment and the scores obtained by video corroborated with the ones made at the bedside (Video 3.1 on Expert Consult).

The scale consists of 11 categories and 15 items, each of which can be rated from a score of 0 up to 4, with a range of 0–42 (Video 3.2 on Expert Consult). The higher the score is, the more severe the stroke symptoms are. A score of 0–4 is suggestive of mild symptoms, 5–23 is moderate to severe, and 24 or more is indicative of a very severe stroke and predicts a poorer outcome. Utilization of this score allows the clinician to assess disease burden, risk-stratify individuals for potential intervention, and prognosticate on patient outcome (Table 3.1).

Table 3.1 National Institute of Health Stroke Scale (NIHSS).

Score	Level of stroke
0	No stroke
1–4	Minor stroke
5–15	Moderate stroke
15–20	Moderate to severe stroke
21–42	Severe stroke

Through video, the examiner is able to score an individual's level of consciousness, orientation, and ability to follow commands. The level of alertness is scored from 0 to 3, depending on the level of stimulation required to maintain patient response to the examiner. Assessment of orientation and patient comprehension is scored based on the response to two questions and following of two specific commands. The patient should always be asked their age and the current month, and instructed to perform eye opening and fist closure. In order to preserve interrater reliability, these two questions and commands have to remain consistent without deviations (Video 3.3 on Expert Consult).

Gaze and extraocular movements can be assessed by having a patient look to the cardinal positions of gaze. A provider may require additional assistance when there is a gaze preference and there is a need to see if this preference can be overcome with vestibular-ocular movements (Video 3.4 on Expert Consult). Visual fields are assessed in each eye with the contralateral eye closed; another set of hands at the bedside at this stage would be helpful but not necessary if the patient is able to alternately close one eye then the other (Video 3.5 on Expert Consult). Facial symmetry requires a close look and requires the camera to be capable of zoom or manually move toward the patient and is a score between 0 and 3; no asymmetry results in a score of 0, while complete facial paralysis, encompassing the upper and lower facial muscles, earns a score of 3 (Video 3.6 on Expert Consult).

The next aspect of the NIHSS is performing the motor exam. The goal is to determine the extent of motor deficits the patient may be experiencing and determine their laterality, thus helping to further localize the stroke clinically. This part of the exam is accomplished by having the patient elevate and extend each arm and leg for a count of 10 and 5, respectively. The arms are in a supinated position and the legs are extended straight at 30 degrees. Strength is scored from 0 to 4. This is easily done via telemedicine with a cooperative patient, but in someone who's consciousness is altered, having an assistant at the bedside can be very helpful. This, person can assist by positioning the limb being tested in an extended position and removing any external support. This will allow the examiner to determine the level of weakness. Each individual limb is tested separately; one extremity at a time. A patient who maintains their arm extended without any appreciable drift receives a score of 0; observable drift without striking the bed earns a score of 1; inability to maintain antigravity and striking the bed is 2; inability to overcome gravity is scored 3; and if no appreciable movement and complete flaccidity is observed, the patient gets the maximum score of 4 (Video 3.7 on Expert Consult).

Items 7–11 are best assessed with bedside assistance. Ataxia is one of the items that varies the most from one examiner to the next. It assesses the coordination and fluidity of movement in the upper and lower extremities by having a patient perform finger to nose and heel to shin movements, respectively. The patient is required to touch the examiner/assistant's finger and then move to touch their nose, and back again. For the lower extremity, the patient is required to rub their shin vertically with the contralateral heel between the ankle and knee. Each extremity is tested. Ataxia is scored if there is poor coordination out of proportion to the weakness. The patient is scored 0 if they are too weak to go through the movements successfully or the amount of incoordination is thought to be reflective and proportionate to their level of weakness. A score of 1 is given if there is poor coordination in one limb and 2 is given for ataxia seen in two limbs (Video 3.8 on Expert Consult).

Sensory evaluation is straightforward and involves assessing the patient's perception of a pinprick. The face, arms, and legs are assessed: a score of 0 is given if no sensory deficits are perceived; 1 is given if the patient is able to sense the pin but the affected side senses it less sharply; and a score of 2 is given for severe sensory loss with no perception of sensation (Video 3.9 on Expert Consult).

For the assessment of speech and language, the NIH provides specific language cards that are used to assess the level of dysarthric speech, aphasia, and possible visual neglect. It is imperative to ensure that the images are clearly visible to the patient and that visual aids such as glasses are used if needed. Consistency is necessary to maintain the reliability of the scoring. The severity of aphasia is scored from 0 to 3. A score of 0 indicates that the patient is without language difficulties and can answer questions, follow commands, and exhibit no anomia or alexia when shown pictures and sentences on the provided language cards. A score of 1 is for mild to moderate language deficits with the patient being understandable the majority of the time. A score of 2 implies that the examiner has poor comprehension of the patient's expressive speech and there could be a receptive component, while 3 indicates global aphasia and mute speech (Video 3.10 on Expert Consult).

The level of dysarthria is assessed by having the patient read or repeat the listed words provided. The level of clarity is scored between 0 and 2, with 0 indicating normal articulation, 1 representing mild slurring with the examiner being able to decipher the majority of the words, and 2 is severe dysarthria, with most of the words uttered being very slurred and unintelligible (Video 3.11 on Expert Consult).

The last section of the exam is the evaluation of neglect with a score from 0 to 2. This could be determined by using information ascertained by the earlier elements of the exam or applying the method of double sensory stimulation simultaneously to both sides and assess for extinction of the patient's perception of the stimulation (Video 3.12 on Expert Consult).

The NIH Stroke Scale has some allowances where certain parts of the exam that are not able to be completed due to physical barriers. Categories 5 and 6 (the motor exam) and Category 10 (dysarthria) are such examples. If the examiner cannot score a patient who has a motor limitation such as a fused or amputated limb, or a patient who is intubated and therefore whose level of speech clarity is not able to be determined, allowances will need to be made. An intubated patient will, however, be scored 3 for aphasia.

When adhered to faithfully, the NIH Stroke Scale is a useful and reliable tool to assess stroke severity and determine the patient's eligibility for a higher level of acute care and intervention. For a complete explanation of the NIH and reference material, you can visit www.nihstrokescale.org.

Despite the new developments in stroke treatments and that the numbers of primary/comprehensive stroke centers increasing each year, there are still areas where stroke specialists are not available. Studies have shown that specialized stroke care is associated with improved outcomes and expedited evaluation for acute treatment and intervention. Telemedicine is able to bridge this potential gap in care and make available the services and expertise of specialties that may not be available to more geographically isolated areas.

Reference

1. www.nihstrokescale.org.

CHAPTER 4

Telemedicine for evaluation of clinical epilepsy

Katherine Noe, MD, PhD
Associate Professor of Neurology, Neurology, Mayo Clinic Arizona, Phoenix, AZ, United States

Introduction

Epilepsy management encompasses a spectrum of disease acuity and locations. Whether providing chronic disease management in the outpatient setting, acute consults in the hospital for new onset or breakthrough seizures, or
critical care management of status epilepticus, there are now opportunities
for this care to occur virtually rather than in-person. Technology to facilitate video-enabled communication between provider and patient has been
available for some time, but use for epilepsy care was limited and largely
restricted to inpatient consultations provided as a component of broader
hospital teleneurology services. The ongoing COVID-19 pandemic has
fostered the rapid embrace of telemedicine for routine outpatient epilepsy
care. While many previous financial and bureaucratic barriers to adoption of
virtual care have been removed, providers must still prepare for the unique
considerations and challenges of seizure management provided remotely.

Opportunities in virtual epilepsy care

Once the current global pandemic is stabilized, it is likely that the demand
for video epilepsy visits will remain high. Convenience has been one obvious benefit described by many telemedicine users. Video visits can offer
greater efficiency than in-person visits, minimizing the need to arrange
time away from work, home, and other activities. Many adults with epilepsy face specific challenges with travel to doctor visits because of the legal
restriction of driving privileges with this diagnosis. In the United States,
people with epilepsy are five times more likely to report transportation as a
barrier to accessing health care than others.[1] Even those who have access to
means of transport in their locale may not have in-person neurologic care
within reach. A 2012 Institute of Medicine report found that close to half of

people living with epilepsy have limited to no access to specialized epilepsy care from a neurologist or epileptologist.[2] This is particularly true in rural and underserved urban areas. Telemedicine offers a means to expand timely access to providers with expertise in seizure management by removing the barrier of physical access to a clinic or hospital. The pool of individuals who would benefit from virtual epilepsy care is even larger when one considers the international market.

Initial epilepsy history and physical examination
Previsit preparation

Just as with in-person clinic visits, adequate previsit preparation can improve both the efficiency and effectiveness of a video consultation. Electronic forms can also be effective for obtaining basic elements of the history, including current medications. Validated screening instruments for common epilepsy comorbidities such as depression can be completed and submitted electronically in advance of the appointment. Furthermore, if the digital platform allows sharing of video clips, patients may be able to obtain a cell phone video capturing representative spells or seizures, which they can show to the provider at the time of the appointment.

The successful virtual consultation

The concerns of taking a comprehensive history from the patient are not significantly different whether the visit is done in person or by telemedicine. When investigating possible seizures, an eyewitness account can often be crucial, particularly when the event involves alteration of awareness or amnesia. During a face-to-face visit, it can be challenging to obtain these accounts, given the burdens of time and effort for a witness to accompany a patient to the doctor's office. Telemedicine platforms may facilitate the participation of friends and family, particularly during times of lockdown, when many family members may be present in the home. For those who are remote from the patient's location, some platforms will allow a unique meeting link to be sent to the eyewitness, allowing them to join the virtual visit for the brief period necessary to provide their account. Some providers may fear that the digital interaction may preclude accurate detection of nonverbal cues to issues ranging from discomfort with the conversation, psychiatric comorbidity, or psychogenic nonepileptic spells. The author's experience has been that these cues are generally similarly detectable on a video visit as they are in the office. The video visit offers an added intimacy of interacting with the patient in their home environment, which may increase patient comfort during the overall interaction. In addition, the laws on driving after a seizure vary from state to state, but the common bond is that the laws limits the patient's ability to get around, even to see their doctor. This barrier is now removed via the use of telemedicine. The previously restricted patient can now see their doctor via a video visit and save the time and potential risk of driving.

The comprehensive neurologic examination that is a standard part of the in-person visit cannot be fully completed virtually in the way we are accustomed to performing it. In particular, assessment in the sensory examination of reflexes, tone, and subtle motor deficits is significantly restricted. However, common concerns regarding the person with epilepsy such as cognitive function, nystagmus, tremor, dysmetria, coordination, and gait instability can be reasonably assessed over a video connection. Virtual examination of the patient's extra-ocular movements by asking the patient to look in each quadrant can be helpful in evaluating for nystagmus. Having the patient extend their arms toward the camera and then point inward toward their nose can assist in evaluating for tremor and dysmetria. Asking the patient to walk in front of the camera will enable you to evaluate for unsteady gait. During the video interview, you can observe for drowsiness, jerky movements, automatisms, or other signs of involuntary motor movements. Examination of the skin can be performed to check for rashes. Asking the patient to show their teeth can be helpful when evaluating patients taking Dilantin, to screen for gingerval hyperplasia. Evidence comparing the effectiveness of in-person versus virtual initial consultations for the evaluation of seizures in epilepsy in regards to accuracy of diagnosis or clinical outcomes is lacking at this time. It is hoped that studies on the effectiveness of virtual consultations for epilepsy will be forthcoming based on rapid widespread adoption of this model in recent months due to COVID-19.

Evaluation and ongoing management

Once patients have an established diagnosis of epilepsy, follow-up care is often focused less on ongoing assessment of changes in physical examination and more on reporting of seizure control and epilepsy comorbidities. For this reason, telemedicine follow-up for this patient population may be particularly appealing. Use of an electronic seizure diary is a simple tool that can be helpful during return visits. In reviewing common testing, radiographic images can be reviewed relatively easily with patients in the virtual environment as long as the platform allows for sharing of digital images. Most providers are already well versed in electronic review of laboratory studies. Considerations for electroencephalography (EEG) in the telemedicine environment are described in a separate chapter. While the results of imaging and EEG can be reviewed virtually, the testing itself requires in-person acquisition. If testing will be performed remotely, consider whether the timeliness and quality will be sufficient for your needs. If not, the patient should be advised in advance of the virtual care visit that they will need to travel to your physical location to complete the comprehensive evaluation. Medication management is much simpler if the system is set up for electronic prescribing, avoiding the need for phone calls to the pharmacy or mailing/faxing paper prescriptions. In-person visits are still needed for programming of epilepsy devices including the vagus nerve stimulator (VNS), responsive neurostimulator (RNS), and deep brain stimulator (DBS).

Although the literature on telemedicine for follow-up epilepsy care is limited, early published experience has been generally positive. A Veterans Administration study of teleneurology services for outpatient management of chronic neurologic conditions including epilepsy in an older, rural patient population found very high patient satisfaction with quality of care and convenience.[3] The office, however, did note some concern of excess emergency department visits compared to what was expected in those receiving virtual care. There was also financial benefit, with 96% of participants reporting that virtual care saved them time and money.[3] Similarly, a small randomized adults with in person ($n = 18$) versus virtual ($n = 23$) follow-up for epilepsy in Canada found that the avoided loss of productivity, travel, and hotel costs resulted in an average saving of $466 Canadian.[4] The majority of those in the study were dependent on others for transportation to in-person visits.[4] Another pilot study for epilepsy telemedicine showed a 50% reduction in no-show rate compared to face-to-face clinic visits, which should translate to cost savings to the medical practice.[5] Finally, a comparison of 155 patients managed via virtual versus in-person visits for epilepsy over a 3-month period found equivalent outcomes for seizure control, emergency room visits, and hospitalizations.[6]

Summary

The growth of virtual care options for people with epilepsy is a welcome transformation. Teleneurology for seizures should help address long-standing barriers to optimal care from limited access to personal transportation and limited availability of specialized epilepsy services affecting many regions. While there are challenges in obtaining a traditional comprehensive neurologic examination compared to in-person interactions, much of the standard seizure assessment can be similarly completed in the virtual environment. There are also advantages to the provider and the patient in terms of efficiency and potentially cost. Assuming that administrative barriers to the provision of virtual care are not reinstated, it is likely that virtual visits will see expanded use in the care of patients with seizures in the near future.

References

1. Thurman DJ, Kobau R, Luo Y-H, Helmers SC, Zack MM. Health-care access among adults with epilepsy: the U.S. National Health Interview Survey, 2010 and 2013. *Epilepsy Behav.* 2016;55:186–188.
2. Institute of Medicine. *Epilepsy Across the Spectrum: Promoting Health and Understanding.* Washington, DC: The National Academies Press; 2012. https://doi.org/10.17226/13379.
3. Davis LE, Harnar J, LaChey-Barbee LA, Richardson SP, Fraser A, King MK. Using teleneurology to deliver chronic neurologic care to rural veterans: analysis of the first 1100 patient visits. *Telemed e-Health.* 2019;25(4):274–278.
4. Ahmed SN, Mann C, Sinclair DB, et al. Feasibility of epilepsy follow-up care through telemedicine: a pilot study on the patient perspective. *Epilepsia.* 2008;49(4):573–585.
5. Haddad N, Grant I, Eswaran H. Telemedicine for patients with epilepsy: a pilot experience. *Epilepsy.* 2015;44:1–4.
6. Rasmussen KA, Hartshorn JC. A comparison of epilepsy patients in a traditional ambulatory clinic and a telemedicine clinic. *Epilepsia.* 2005;46:767–770.

CHAPTER 5

The ophthalmologic exam

Garvin Davis, MD, MPH
Director, Retinal Disease and Surgery, The Robert Cizik Eye Clinic, Houston, TX, United States

Introduction

A comprehensive ophthalmic exam can be critical to the diagnosis and management of neurological conditions. Composed of eight different parts, certain components of a complete ophthalmic exam are easily adapted to telemedicine and others are quite challenging. In this chapter, we will discuss the current options available to the clinician as it relates to examining the eye, current practices, and future adaptions specific to ophthalmology.

Telemedicine can be broadly divided into two broad categories: asynchronous (data are collected and discussed at a later time) and synchronous (data are exchanged in real time).[1] We will discuss asynchronous telemedicine in what the author refers to as the hybrid model of ophthalmology. Historically the hybrid model has been the one most often applied to ophthalmology.

Patient selection

The physician and practice should select patients appropriate for telemedicine visits based on objective clinical criteria (e.g., established vs. new patients, age)[1] and subjective patient-specific criteria such as ability to access and use technology. Some physicians find that establishing relationships with new patients is more difficult than maintaining or following up chronic conditions using telemedicine.

Scheduling visits

Telemedicine visits can either be scheduled as a separate clinic or integrated into a traditional clinic. In ophthalmology, the average dilated patient exam lasts 1.5 h, whereas the average nondilated patient exam lasts 30 min. Synchronous and asynchronous telemedicine exams usually only require 15–20 min of physician and patient time, given that dilation is often not possible. Many of the time-consuming aspects of the exam have already been completed.

Prior to the day of the visit, staff members send the patient information about how to prepare for the telemedicine visit through electronic mail (email), phone call, or secure messaging. Consent for the visit is obtained verbally and documented in the electronic health record (EHR), or some telemedicine software programs include consent. The patient is asked to test the internet connection and their device's compatibility with the software solution that will be used. Virtual visits can be converted to a telephone call if there are technological problems on either side during the call.

Software and hardware technology solutions

Often the physician will have a separate telemedicine software platform that allows for a secure HIPAA-compliant system that allows the physician to schedule patients, interact through video conferencing, and share screens. The physician will also have a separate EHR system that is most often used for in-person visits.

Internet bandwidth and computers with sufficient processing speed are essential to a high-quality telemedicine visit. Many physicians also find it more helpful to use large screens to visualize the patient rather than small devices such as a cell phone or tablet.[2]

The traditional ophthalmic exam

Technicians will often perform a standard medical interview and gather details of the patient's chief complaint, history of present illness, past medical history, past ocular history, surgical history, current medications, allergies, family history, social history, and review of systems. This can be done either prior to the virtual visit or during the visit. Once this information is recorded in the medical record, the physician may embark upon a specific ophthalmologic exam that consists of:
- visual acuity, near and far, with and without glasses;
- pupil exam;
- ocular motility;
- . visual field;
- intraocular pressure;

- external exam (eyelids and globe position in the orbit);
- anterior segment exam; and
- fundus or retina exam.

With a cooperative patient in a well-equipped ophthalmic office, the exam is often completed quickly and efficiently, usually including the 20-min dilation time needed to examine the fundus adequately. Most often the exam requires many pieces of specialized equipment, including:

- phoropter to refract and find the best corrected vision;
- bright focused light to test the pupils;
- tonometer to test intraocular pressure;
- slit lamp to examine the translucent structures of the front of the eye: cornea, anterior chamber, lens, and anterior vitreous; and
- direct or indirect (more commonly) ophthalmoscope for dilated fundus exam (Fig. 5.1).

Often ophthalmologists will use very specialized machines in the office to:

- formally standardize and quantify visual fields;
- photograph the optic nerve and fundus through either undilated or dilated pupil;
- measure the retina nerve fiber layer or the retina layers and fovea via optical coherence tomography;
- carry out fluorescein angiography to evaluate the perfusion of the retina; or
- evaluate the shape of the cornea and topography.

There are many textbooks that carefully explain traditional methods of ocular exam. Here, we will explore each major part of the ocular exam and consider adaptations for telemedicine.

Visual acuity

There are several mobile applications and online tools that can be used to check the patient's visual acuity and refraction, as well as other visual tests. One example is the Eye Handbook, which allows the patient to test visual acuity, color vision, and contrast sensitivity, and which contains an Amsler grid. The physician can use other tools included in the application such as an OKN drum, fluorescein light, and fixation targets to examine the patient synchronously (see Fig. 5.2).

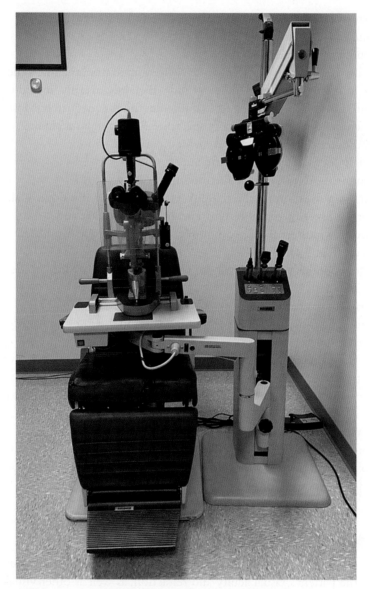

Fig. 5.1 Ophthalmology exam chair with slit lamp and phoropter.

These tools have not been validated in the remote clinical setting and are not as accurate as in-office testing, as they rely on the patient's subjective cooperation. The method of testing visual acuity will certainly change if the patient returns to the office. Trends can be observed, however, if the same methodology is used for subsequent visits and exams.

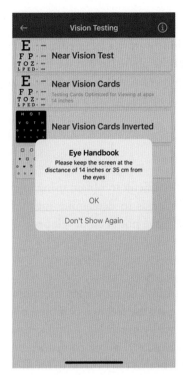
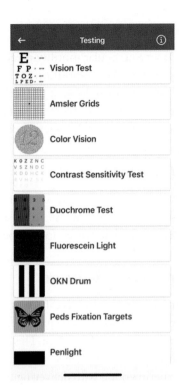

Fig. 5.2 Screenshot of Eye Handbook developed by Cloud Nine Development.

Pupil exam

Examination of the pupils tests the afferent system of the visual system. Traditionally this exam is carried out in a dim room with the swinging flashlight test. The physician first notes the size of each pupil in dim light. Normally the pupils are the same size and approximately 5 mm in diameter. A bright light is shone into one eye and then swung to the other. The direct and consensual responses are noted. The presence of a relative afferent pupil defect denotes a difference in the afferent pathway.

Using telemedicine, the physician can have a companion assist the patient or have the patient arrange the video camera and light such that the physician can observe the pupils. This is best performed by having the patient face the camera and the companion swing a bright flashlight from behind the camera position. It may be difficult to determine accurately a mild RAPD and/or distinguish the changes from near accommodation; however, a significant RAPD will be able to be observed.

Ocular motility

Observing ocular motility is relatively straightforward via telemedicine. The patient is asked to position the camera so that the physician can see the eyes. The patient can look at the screen and the physician will ask the patient to follow a target in the traditional H pattern, looking for defects in cranial nerves III, IV, and VI. Please see video.

Visual field

Accurate objective measures of visual field are difficult to obtain using telemedicine. One can use tools such as Amsler grids to determine measure central field; however, formal perimetry tools have not been developed.

Intraocular pressure

Intraocular pressure is difficult to measure virtually. The most basic method is to ask the patient to palpate their eye and compare the feel to a common object such as a piece of fruit. This method is inherently unreliable, as studies have shown that inexperienced clinicians are not accurate.[3,4] Some companies are experimenting with delivering tools to the patient that can be used to measure intraocular pressure at home such as the iCare Tonometer and the Sensimed Triggerfish contact lens. These devices are expensive, and studies have shown that patient training can be difficult[5] and the results difficult to interpret.[6]

External exam (eyelids and globe position in the orbit)

Positioning the camera with appropriate lighting makes the observation of the external exam straightforward.

Anterior segment exam

Technology does not currently exist that enables the patient to allow the physician to perform a formal slit lamp exam synchronously. A basic penlight exam can be performed, however.

Fundus or retina exam

Examining the retina or optic nerve is not easily done during a synchronous visit. Although the cameras on phones and tablets can be adapted to image the retina and have been proven effective, devices that allow the patient to self-image have not been developed for use at home.[7,8] Technology does exist to image the retina in a small format, however. Mobile fundus cameras that the patient can hold themselves, such as the Welch Allyn RetinaVue 700 Imager, allow for high-resolution images suitable for diagnosing diabetic retinopathy, macular degeneration, and optic neuropathy.[9] However, these technologies are very expensive and would likely only be feasible in a clinical model where many patients can borrow the same device.

The hybrid telemedicine model

In an asynchronous or hybrid telemedicine model, the patient is asked to come to the office or an imaging center for testing prior to a follow-up telemedicine visit with the physician. This allows the patient to avoid spending time in the waiting room to see the doctor. Ideally the patient will be scheduled to come into the office and only see a photographer. The photographer can perform any number of tests including optical coherence tomography, fundus photography, fluorescein photography, or formal visual field testing. The physician will then arrange to have another call with the patient to review the tests and discuss diagnosis and treatment.

Home monitoring

The ForSee home monitoring device (NotalVision) was developed in 2010 to allow patients with macular disease to monitor for changes in the central 10° visual field. There are also visual discrimination applications such as mVT (Vital Art and Science) that perform similar functions.

Conclusion

Given the benefits of telemedicine (less exposure to other patients, less expensive visits, convenience), several physicians are using technology to examine patients. The pandemic has elevated the patient's awareness of the possible technologies, and with the techniques above, a sufficient ophthalmic exam can be performed effectively and efficiently.

References

1. Areaux RG, Campomanes AGDA, Indaram M, Shah AS, Consortium PT-O. Your eye doctor will virtually see you now: synchronous patient-to-provider virtual visits in pediatric tele-ophthalmology. *J AAPOS.* 2020. https://doi.org/10.1016/j.jaapos.2020.06.004.

2. Saleem SM, Pasquale LR, Sidoti PA, Tsai JC. Virtual ophthalmology: telemedicine in a COVID-19 era. *Am J Ophthalmol.* 2020;216:237–242.
3. Baum J, Chaturvedi N, Netland PA, Dreyer EB. Assessment of intraocular pressure by palpation. *Am J Ophthalmol.* 1995;119:650–651.
4. Birnbach CD, Leen MM. Digital palpation of intraocular pressure. *Ophthalmic Surg Lasers.* 1998;29:754–757.
5. McGarva E, Farr J, Dabasia P, Lawrenson JG, Murdoch IE. Initial experience in self-monitoring of intraocular pressure. *Eur J Ophthalmol.* 2020. https://doi.org/10.1177/1120672120920217, 112067212092021.
6. Huang J, Phu J, Kalloniatis M, Zangerl B. Determining significant elevation of intraocular pressure using self-tonometry. *Optom Vis Sci.* 2020;97:86–93.
7. Khanamiri HN, Nakatsuka A, El-Annan J. Smartphone fundus photography. *J Vis Exp.* 2017;55:958. https://doi.org/10.3791/55958.
8. Mohammadpour M, Heidari Z, Mirghorbani M, Hashemi H. Smartphones, tele-ophthalmology, and VISION 2020. *Int J Ophthalmol.* 2017;10:1909–1918.
9. Stebbins K. Diabetic retinal examinations in frontline care using retinavue care delivery model. *Point Care.* 2019;18:37–39.

CHAPTER 6

Neuro-ophthalmology evaluation

Stacy V. Smith, MD
Neuro-Ophthalmologist, Houston Methodist Neurological Institute and Blanton Eye Institute, Woodlands, TX, United States

Introduction

As technological advances allow greater virtual connectivity for many aspects of business and social life, the medical field is also developing innovative ways to extend our care. Certain specialties lend themselves more easily to this form of care. Neuro-ophthalmology relies heavily on in-person physical exam with specialized equipment and diagnostic testing that cannot be fully replicated in the home setting. Yet, some providers use a combination of telehealth applications and remote review of locally performed exams and imaging to provide care to patients in rural or underserved areas. The recent pandemic spurred further development and widespread utilization of new methods to evaluate and treat patients while minimizing face-to-face contact. According to a May 2020 survey of neuro-ophthalmologists' telehealth use, video visit use increased from about 4% to 68% as a way to maintain patient care during the pandemic.[1] Maintaining an appropriate standard of care must be balanced against our Hippocratic oath, particularly "first, do no harm." Many neuro-ophthalmology patients have comorbid conditions that place them at high risk of morbidity or mortality with COVID-19 infection. In addition, a delay in care may lead to permanent vision loss and disability. As community home quarantine orders and patient fears of contracting COVID-19 impact patient presentation to clinic for initial and follow-up evaluations, use of telehealth technology can help maintain a relationship with these patients that is essential to their long-term well-being.[2]

Preparing for a telehealth visit

Prior to initiating a teleneuro-ophthalmology evaluation, it is important to screen patients for appropriateness. The first step is a practical evaluation to ensure a patient can participate in a telehealth exam. Patients must provide consent to participate in a telehealth visit, and basic internet and/ or telephone service is necessary to provide a synchronous connection between the patient and physician. While smartphones, laptops, and tablets are relatively common household items, not all patients have such a device available to them. Furthermore, some patients may not be comfortable using the necessary technology including the virtual visit platform and exam applications. It may be helpful to have a family member or friend present as a support person to help patients set up for a visit and to assist with certain portions of the exam during the visit.

Reviewing prior records and imaging allows the provider to triage patients for urgency as well as appropriate visit type. Efferent disorders typically have external signs in the pupil, eye, and lid movements that can be evaluated via video. Many afferent visual and sensory complaints can also be evaluated by a telehealth visit with supplemental exam and imaging information from a recent evaluation.[3] In a survey of telehealth adoption by neuro-ophthalmologists, many providers reported that video visits can be helpful in the evaluation of cranial nerve palsies, migraine with aura, positive visual phenomenon, anisocoria, binocular diplopia, ocular myasthenia gravis, ptosis, and transient visual loss. With supporting imaging such as fundus photos, ocular coherence tomography, magnetic resonance imaging, and visual fields, one may also be able to evaluate optic neuritis, pituitary tumors, idiopathic intracranial hypertension, and certain eye pain complaints. Due to the variable nature of disorders such as myasthenia gravis, one often has to rely entirely on the history, as in-person exam may be completely unrevealing. Optic neuritis and temporal arteritis both have pain as a feature. The provider can evaluate this pain further during a remote exam by having the patient perform eye movements and/or palpate their own temples. The survey found that most respondents did not find video visits helpful for evaluation of nonarteritic anterior ischemic optic neuropathy, possible arteritic ischemic optic neuropathy, and optic atrophy.[1] These conditions often require frequent fundus exams for monitoring. Recent records and use of the tools described later in the chapter can support a partial evaluation via telehealth until the patient can present to clinic for any neuro-ophthalmology concern. An initial telehealth visit may help one further triage the urgency of this in-person exam.

There are multiple types of telehealth visits that a provider can utilize for patient care. A real-time synchronous video visit is the closest to an in-person visit, as it allows for a history as well as a limited exam. While the standard face-to-face visit allows more natural interaction with the patient using subtle facial and body language cues, the current need for mask use by both patients and providers hampers this to a degree. In this way, use of video can be a superior method for safely interacting without masks until social distancing measures end. Telephone visits consist of synchronous verbal communication only. They are well suited for counseling established patients on test results and disease management. In instances where an in-person physical exam is necessary, the provider can perform a history via video or telephone to minimize time spent in direct contact.[4]

Asynchronous telehealth consists of patients submitting symptom updates, videos, and/or images via a patient portal or other secure communication to the provider for review at another time. While asynchronous telehealth is most commonly used for established patients, some facilities offer second opinion evaluations for patients, which consist of an expert reviewing a set of records and providing a written report of their assessment, as well as answers to a set of questions submitted by the patient. If a patient consents, a referring provider can initiate an interprofessional consultation. The consulting provider reviews the records and provides a verbal and/or written report to the referring provider without ever interacting with the patient.[4]

The virtual visit

History

The neuro-ophthalmology history is key to building a differential diagnosis. The history helps establish whether the visual disturbance is acute or chronic, stable or progressive, monocular or binocular, and painful or painless. One can also elucidate any other associated neurological or systemic symptoms. The patient can relate symptom onset and progression, subjective symptoms such as pain that we cannot objectively observe, and variable symptoms that may not be present at the time of evaluation. A history can always be documented for any visit type, but the level of detail and patient input varies. Even for asynchronous visits, patients can complete a history questionnaire and/or free text summary of their complaint for the physician.

Indirect history can come from the consulting provider, family, and review of records, which are often just as valuable as the patient's account. Prior eye exam records help to establish baseline vision, when the ophthalmic changes started, and how they have progressed over time. This is particularly helpful in asymptomatic patients found to have significant pathology identified on routine exam. The complexity of the visual and neurological systems makes it difficult for some patients to describe their experience accurately. For instance, a person may not recognize vision loss until it reaches a certain threshold, or until they attempt to view monocularly with a non-dominant eye. This "sudden realization" can seem like "sudden onset" to a patient. Patients may also confuse vision loss in one eye with loss of part of the visual field in both eyes. The term "double vision" may be used by patients experiencing blurry vision or another visual disturbance. Obtaining ancillary information from family may also help, particularly if the vision change impacts self-care, driving, or other routine tasks.

Physical exam

The greatest challenge to virtual neuro-ophthalmology visits is the exam. A virtual neuro-ophthalmology visit is not possible with current technology, but many exam components can be adapted to video evaluation and/or approximated with validated applications for the computer, tablet, or smartphone. If the referring optometry or ophthalmology provider evaluated the patient in person, they may be able to provide further support in the way of examination findings and diagnostic imaging. We will review remote evaluation options for each exam component. The physician can complete as much of the exam as possible virtually, and then have the patient complete any remaining components in-person on the same day or at a later date.

Visual acuity is the sharpness of vision, typically assessed by reading a chart of numbers or letters at a set distance. Loss of acuity can occur with pathology in various parts of the eye, including damage to the optic nerve. In the clinic setting, this is performed by a technician or the physician and may include use of lenses and instruments to correct refractive errors. A variety of tools exist for home assessment of visual acuity. Patients can print a vision card, or use a validated visual acuity application. Validated applications include PEEK Acuity, Visual Acuity XL, Vision@home, and Eye Cart Pro. A near-vision test card can be accessed at https://farsight.care (Table 6.1).[4,5-9]

Color vision is the ability to discern differences in wavelength. Changes in color vision can be an early or subtle indicator of optic neuropathy. Color vision testing can be assessed by presenting the color plate or color cards on the video, but this is limited by resolution and screen color displays. The Eye Handbook app was validated in comparison to the Ishihara color vision test.[4,10]

The visual field is the area each eye can see, typically assessed in primary gaze with the eyes directed straight ahead. This is particularly help in neuro-ophthalmology for localization of a lesion along the visual pathway. In the clinic, automated perimetry and direct confrontation are used. The

Table 6.1 Telemedicine tools.[4–13]

Exam component	Application/website	Device compatibility
Visual acuity (requires assistance for distance vision testing)	PEEK Acuity	Android
	Visual Acuity XL	iPad
	Vision@home	iPhone, Android
	Eye Chart Pro	iPad
	https://farsight.care	Computer
Color vision	Eye Handbook	iPhone, Android
Visual field	MRF Glaucoma	iPad
	www.eyesimplify.com	Computer

referring provider may be able to provide recent testing for your interpretation. The MRF Glaucoma Lite application for Apple iPads provides reliable remote visual field testing according to several trials. The same technology can be accessed on a computer browser at www.eyesimplify.com.[4,11–13]

Pupil size, symmetry, and reactivity provide details on optic nerve function. Anisocoria may indicate autonomic innervation deficits. The exam includes observation of both pupils in light and dark, with accommodation, and while slowly swinging the flashlight back and forth between the eye to detect a relative afferent pupillary defect (RAPD). It is important to note that in many optometry and general ophthalmology practices, the pupils are evaluated by a technician and the patient receives dilating drops before the physician evaluates them. Therefore, the neuro-ophthalmologist always personally confirms this exam component because the records may be unreliable. When performing this exam by video, the physician can instruct a support person on how to move a small flashlight while the provider observes the video. One can also evaluate RAPD in ambient lighting by having the patient covering one eye at a time while the examiner observes the uncovered pupil. Since the pupils should be equal in size, a larger pupil in one eye suggests an RAPD.

Extraocular motor movement and eye alignment are assessed in each of the cardinal gaze directions. A patient can follow commands via video to demonstrate these movements. Ask the patient if there is any pain with the movement. If diplopia is present but eye deviation is not clear, instruct the patient (or support person) in cover testing. The physician can observe while the patient slowly covers and uncovers each eye. They can then observe while the patient moves their hand back and forth from eye to eye for cross-cover testing. Prisms and Maddox rods are helpful in further localizing and precisely measuring abnormal eye position. The patient could then come to the clinic for this next step in evaluation. Similarly, one can assess for proptosis by viewing the patient directly and in profile on the video, followed later by measurement with exophthalmometry in person. Video also allows for observation of the eyelid for ptosis, retraction, lag, fatiguability, and response to rest and ice packs. If possible, have a support person hold up and move a finger target for these tests while the physician observes via video. The provider can also instruct the patient and/or support person in palpation of the temporal arteries, scalp, and trochlear notch.

The anterior segment is normally evaluated by slit lamp. When evaluating a patient remotely, video or photographs can allow for limited assessment of eye appearance, including conjunctival injection and periorbital edema. Additional important elements of the exam that cannot be completed at home include intraocular pressure (IOP) measurement and the fundus exam. Recent records can provide information regarding the IOP. Fundus photos from the referring provider may also allow for limited evaluation of the posterior segment. A virtual visit can help the physician to determine urgency of presentation to the clinic for further slit lamp and fundoscopic examination.

Management: Counseling and treatment

Telehealth lends itself well to the counseling portion of clinical care. Providers can educate patients and answer any questions via video, telephone, and written communication. Patients utilizing telehealth technology can access the North American Neuro-Ophthalmology Society patient educational materials on their website (www.nanosweb.org). Providers can send any prescriptions directly to the pharmacy for the patient, and some pharmacies can then mail the medication to the patient's home. Similarly, the physician can send orders for radiology or laboratory testing to the patient's preferred facility.

Conclusion

While the pandemic has disrupted many aspects of society, it has led to innovation of medical practice. The rapid expansion of telehealth services has allowed physicians to maintain care during social distancing measures, but likely will remain a significant part of health care practice postpandemic. The in-person exam will always be an important part of medicine, but virtual visits may play an increased role in follow-up care. Some predict that hybrid visits of a physician virtual visit combined with in-office exam and testing may become a way to improve access to neuro-ophthalmological care.[14]

Applications and web-based exam tools continue to evolve for remote patient evaluation, which will support underserved and mobility-limited patient populations even after social distancing measures end.

References

1. Moss HE, Lai KE, Ko MW. Survey of telehealth adoption by neuro-ophthalmologists during the COVID-19 pandemic: benefits, barriers and utility. *J Neuroophthalmol.* 2020;40(3):346–355.
2. Ko MW, Busis NA. Tele-neuro-ophthalmology: vision for 20/20 and beyond. *J Neuroophthalmol.* 2020;40(3):378–384.
3. Lai KE, Mackay DD, Ko MW. Teleneuro-ophthalmology. *Pract Neurol.* 2020;40–41. 49, 54.
4. Lai KE, Ko MW, Rucker JC, et al. Tele-neuro-ophthalmology during the age of COVID-19. *J Neuroophthalmol.* 2020;40(3):292–304.
5. Bastawrous A, Rono HK, Livingstone IAT, et al. Development and validation of a smartphone-based visual acuity test (peek acuity) for clinical practice and community-based fieldwork. *JAMA Ophthalmol.* 2015;133(8):930–937.
6. Brady CJ, Eghrari AO, Labrique AB. Smartphone-based visual acuity measurement for screening and clinical assessment. *JAMA.* 2015;314(24):2682–2683.
7. Han X, Scheetz J, Keel S, et al. Development and validation of a smartphone-based visual acuity test (vision at home). *Transl Vis Sci Technol.* 2019;8(4):27.
8. O'Neill S, McAndrew DJ. The validity of visual acuity assessment using mobile technology devices in the primary care setting. *Aust Fam Physician.* 2016;45(4):212–215.
9. Black JM, Jacobs RJ, Phillips G, et al. An assessment of the iPad as a testing platform for distance visual acuity in adults. *BMJ Open.* 2013;3(6), e002730.
10. Ozgur OK, Emborgo TS, Vieyra MB, Huselid RF, Banik R. Validity and acceptance of color vision testing on smartphones. *J Neuroophthalmol.* 2018;38(1):13–16.
11. Schultz AM, Graham EC, You YY, Klistomer A, Graham SL. Performance of iPad-based threshold perimetry in glaucoma and controls. *Clin Exp Ophthalmol.* 2018;46(4):346–355.
12. Kong YXG, He M, Crowston JG, Vingrys AJ. A comparison of perimetric results from a tablet perimeter and Humphrey field analyzer in glaucoma patients. *Transl Vis Sci Technol.* 2016;5(6):2.
13. Prea SM, Kong YXG, Mehta A, et al. Six-month longitudinal comparison of a portable tablet perimeter with the Humphrey field analyzer. *Am J Ophthalmol.* 2018;190:9–16.
14. Grossman SN, Calix R, Tow S, et al. Neuro-ophthalmology in the era of COVID-19: future implications of a public health crisis. *Ophthalmology.* 2020;127(9):e72–e74.

CHAPTER 7

Teleneurology for Parkinson's disease and movement disorders in the COVID-19 pandemic

Zoltan Mari, MD, FAAN[a,b,c,d]

[a]Ruvo Family Chair, Lou Ruvo Center for Brain Health, Neurological Institute, Cleveland Clinic, Las Vegas, NV, United States
[b]Director of Parkinson's & Movement Disorder Program, Lou Ruvo Center for Brain Health, Neurological Institute, Cleveland Clinic, Las Vegas, NV, United States
[c]Adjunct Associate Professor, Neurology, Johns Hopkins University, Baltimore, MD, United States
[d]Clinical Professor, Medicine (Neurology), University of Nevada Las Vegas, Las Vegas, NV, United States

Introduction

Since its branching from internal medicine few decades ago, of which neurology once was a subspecialty itself, subspecialization of neurology has been marching forward at a great pace. As a result, today there are more than two dozen neurology subspecialties[1] and up to three-quarters of graduating neurology residents continue to complete a clinical fellowship program in one of those subspecialties.[2] One of those subspecialties is movement disorders. The term "movement disorders" in general use pertains to "Parkinson's disease, related neurodegenerative and neurodevelopmental disorders, hyperkinetic movement disorders, and abnormalities in muscle tone and motor control",[3] and includes diseases such as dystonia, chorea, ataxia, Tourette syndrome, essential tremor, myoclonus, restless legs syndrome, and many others. While its subspecialty training curriculum is not currently stipulated by the Accreditation Council for Graduate Medical Education and thus movement disorder fellowship programs are not accredited like many others, the several dozen available clinical fellowship programs are usually formal and curriculum-based.[4]

Parkinson's disease (PD), arguably the most important movement disorder, is historically recognized via its four cardinal motor features (resting tremor, bradykinesia, rigidity, and postural instability) and played a pivotal role in the birth of "movement" disorder as a subspecialty field, due to its most recognized features related to impaired movements and motor control.[5] Considering the importance of phenomenology of movement abnormalities, visual observation plays a fundamental role in diagnosing and managing patients with PD and other movement disorders. Therefore, videotaping and video evaluations have become an inevitable part of movement disorder care.[6] It naturally follows that video or "virtual" visits, a pinnacle of telehealth, which allow such visual observation and examination of motor symptoms in movement disorders, represent a care delivery particularly relevant and appropriate in the care of movement disorder patients. Care in PD, relying on the use of virtual visits, was found to be noninferior in comparison to traditional care,[7] including patient and provider satisfaction.[8] Besides PD, telemedicine has been also used for hyperkinetic movement disorders[9] and a wide range of other movement disorders including atypical parkinsonian syndromes,[10] Huntington's disease,[11] and essential tremor.[8]

In addition to the importance of video assessments (which can be technically done via virtual visits), objective measurements in PD and movement disorders, many of which technically and feasibly doable remotely, have been increasingly introduced in PD and movement disorder care. More recently, a new term, "digital phenotyping," has been proposed to describe this novel domain of objective assessment of symptoms and findings in PD and movement disorders.[12] Digital phenotyping represents a novel, critically important direction in the assessment and management of PD and movement disorders, considering its many advantages over traditional care: objectivity, lack of intra- and interrater variability, high reproducibility, feasibility of remote application, ecological validity, higher accuracy and finer grading compared to scales forcing scores into fewer, cruder, arbitrarily defined categories, and often a greater degree of automation.[12]

The year 2020 witnessed unprecedented changes in Parkinson's and movement disorder telehealth practices around the world due to the profound impact of the COVID-19 pandemic.[13] Thanks to the many regulatory adjustments and easing, telehealth access have improved considerably since the start of the pandemic, with many of the financial and regulatory burdens having been eased significantly in no small part due to the CARES Act in the United States.[14]

Deep brain stimulation (DBS) implants have been critical in the management of many movement disorder patients, most notably those with advanced and/or intractable PD, dystonia, and essential tremor (ET). The COVID-19 pandemic profoundly impacted DBS care.[15–17] In addition, a recent survey (2020) has been conducted by the Motor Working Group of the Parkinson Study Group (PSG) in the United States on the impact of COVID-19 on clinical care, clinical research, and advanced therapy (such as

DBS) practice adjustments among movement disorder specialists, and this work has been submitted as an abstract for the 2021 AAN Annual Meeting.

Telemedicine in your movement disorder practice

Due to the profound impact of the COVID-19 pandemic on PD and movement disorder care around the globe,[13,18] movement disorder clinics have witnessed unforeseen, dramatic adjustments in their practices.[13] A number of high-quality editorials have been authored in recent months on the topic.[17,19–22] While many advantages of telemedicine in PD and movement disorders were established well before the pandemic,[20,23,24] including but not limited to feasibility in the age of the internet, cost effectivity (saving travel cost and time, especially when traveling a distance, parking), convenience (especially for those challenged physically in their mobility), high favorability ratings by providers, and satisfaction by patients, the pandemic directed our attention to another major advantage of telehealth delivery of care: eliminating physical contact and thereby risk of viral spread.

Before a detailed practical review of the steps to set up a movement disorder telemedicine practice, it is necessary to review the various modalities and types of telemedicine care. The word "telemedicine" is commonly used in reference to remote synchronous video visits, sometimes also referred to as "virtual visits," during which the patient and the provider are video conferencing in real time. However, there are many other types and options that are included under "telemedicine" in addition to just virtual visits, although undoubtedly this is the most frequent and most widely recognized form of telemedicine. During virtual visits, it is possible to take history, involve a care partner, and a limited motor exam is also usually possible. Some movement disorder scales have been validated for remote use, including a modified version of the Unified Parkinson's Disease Rating Scale[25] and the Unified Huntington's Disease Rating Scale.[11]

While "synchronous" virtual visits are the norm when broadband internet connection is available at both the provider's and the patient's end, so-called "asynchronous" video visits may be considered under certain circumstances, especially in technologically less advanced regions with lack of high-speed internet access. In asynchronous video visits, the patient's examination is recorded—for example, following instructions to include specific tasks or views; it is then uploaded over a low-speed internet connection to a dedicated secure server, from where the provider can access the video recording and evaluate or rate it according to a predetermined protocol.

In addition to synchronous and asynchronous video visits, "telemedicine" in movement disorders may refer to visits involving interdisciplinary care,[23] the use of objective devices[12] such as wearables or "telemetry," tele-psychiatry and tele-therapy, management of advanced therapies such as DBS[17], and screening for advanced therapies and research eligibility.

The international Movement Disorders Society (MDS), through its Telemedicine Study Group,[26] has developed a step-by-step guide[27] for providers to set up or optimize their telemedicine practice specifically for Parkinson's disease and movement disorders. A webinar, with a similar goal and also granting continuing medical education credits, was published by the same Telemedicine Study Group.[28]

Before beginning to set up a telemedicine practice and delve into any telemedicine technical steps and guidance to any depth, it is important to review and fully understand the specific national, regional, local, and (if applicable) institutional regulatory environment of one's practice, as it pertains to providing telehealth care. Specific regulations across countries and regions may vary widely. The MDS Telemedicine Study Group has compiled an extensive database that is available online and is updated regularly to aid movement disorder providers with their review of regional regulatory information.[29] A detailed review of telemedicine regulatory status was also included in a peer-reviewed publication by the same group.[13]

In addition to regulatory requirements, it is critical to address the financial aspects and feasibility of a telemedicine practice. Naturally, this varies greatly by regions and countries.[13] In the United States the most comprehensive review of nonface-to-face evaluation and management codes have been prepared by the American Academy of Neurology.[30] It is believed that telehealth may become part of an integrated and patient-centered management model in PD, where tangible, validated, and relevant health outcomes,[31] as opposed to fee-for-service incentives, will primarily determine health care practices, as is predominantly the case currently in the United States.

After applicable regulatory requirements and billing/coding information have been reviewed and complied with, the next challenge in telemedicine setup is securing the necessary hardware and software. Fortunately, most modern medical offices nowadays either are already equipped or can easily be furnished with the basic hardware needed for a telemedicine setup, including a computer or other device that is outfitted with audio and video capabilities and a broadband internet connection.[27,28] Typical devices may include a desktop or laptop computer, a tablet or cell phone, with camera, microphone, and speakers. A somewhat more complex question is the choice of software. Increasingly, some electronic medical record (EMR) systems include built-in video visit capability. It is necessary to confirm if such an option is available or another preferred platform is otherwise offered at the practice location, where a provider seeks to begin virtual visits. Fig. 7.1 provides an overview of the relevant decision points usually applicable to most practice environments.

When reviewing software options, especially in cases when these are not already available institutionally or embedded in EMR, privacy is an utmost consideration. While some regulatory agencies and institutions have relaxed the rigor of privacy enforcements in response to the COVID-19 pandemic,[13] the prolongation of the pandemic and widespread adoption and integration of telemedicine led to its normalization, where the rigor of enforcing privacy policies gradually return to their prepandemic baseline.

Once the regulatory and hardware/software matters have been addressed, the next important aspect of setting up a telemedicine practice or, if we want to stay narrow in our definitions as discussed above, virtual visits, will be the proper way of preparing the video and room setup. Tables 7.1A and 7.1B review some steps that can help, for both the provider's (Table 7.1A) and the patient's (Table 7.1B) side. Review the steps outlined in Table 7.2 on how to conduct a teleneurology visit.

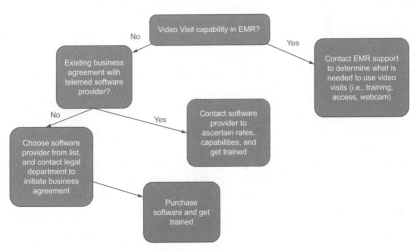

Fig. 7.1 Overview of the telemedicine software selection process.

Table 7.1A Steps to prepare a video and room setup ideally (provider's side).

Background:
- Ensure the area is neat. Limit clutter in the field of view of the camera.
- Avoid shiny surfaces (glass) reflecting light.
- Consider a solid color backdrop ~1 m from camera.

Lighting:
- Ensure face is well lit.
- Sit with a light source in front of your face (e.g., desk lamp, window)—consider two light sources to avoid excessive shadows.
- Close window shades or otherwise block a light source behind you to avoid backlighting.
- Avoid overexposure.
- Some LED lights may flicker in cameras. Try to change lighting (nonflicker LED lights), location, or camera.

Examiner Appearance:
- Use picture-in-picture (show image) to verify your face is centered and close enough to the camera, while capturing hands for gesturing and communication.
- Wear solid-colored clothing; avoid busy patterns.
- Wear a white coat and/or name badge, if this is your regular dress code.
- Ensure intermittent eye contact with the patient by looking at the camera instead of the screen.
- Stand/sit upright (avoid slouching and swiveling the chair; the chair backrest should be lower than shoulder height).
- Don't touch your face (COVID-19!).

Table 7.1B Instructions to send to patients to help prepare their end of a virtual visit.

In the Patient's Home:
- Have a second person available for assistance with video.
- Position seat 2–3 ft from the webcam.
- Place a second seat 8–10 ft from the webcam for full body and gait exam; consider hallway for gait exam.
- Close shades, blinds, and doors to prevent backlighting, and sit facing a light rather than in front of one.
- Limit background clutter, reflection (pictures, mirrors, and windows), and noise (turn off TV, radio).
- Recommend using picture-in-picture in your video software.
- Include a disclaimer if applicable (e.g., the patient provides verbal consent; sign consent acknowledging they have a choice between telemedicine and office care; inform them that the visit is not recorded).

If the Patient is at a Remote Healthcare Site:
- Consider using a telepresenter. These are trained personnel who can assist in portions of the exam that are difficult to perform remotely (e.g., checking tone, pull-test, reflexes, eye movements).
- Examiners should consider the cost of training and having telepresenters available.

Table 7.2 Conducting a teleneurology visit.

- Schedule extra time for troubleshooting.
- Prepare patient expectations:
  - Education before the visit, including review of written materials on telehealth in general and the upcoming visit in particular – a brief educational video or slides explaining the process maybe considered.
  - Allow for possibility of technical difficulties, and backup plan (see next slide); most technical glitches are easily fixed and unlikely to recur.
  - Emphasize ease of rescheduling.
- Do a test run:
  - If possible, ask a staff member to perform a test connection or "trial run" with the patient prior to the scheduled visit. Some software platforms allow testing.
  - If this is not possible, a telephone call reminder, with explanations of what to expect, how to be prepared, and room setup can be helpful.
- If you do not have available IT support, consider a mock visit as the patient, to see the steps the patient will go through to connect.
- Ensure that the patient has a telephone available for the visit.
- Have a backup plan in place (e.g., if an emergency occurs during visit, or for troubleshooting).
- Consider a telephone visit as part of a backup plan.
- Telephone visits can also help triage patients, and assist patients who may not have access to telemedicine.
- The patient may be anxious about the technological aspects of the visit— remember to start with a friendly introduction to help put him/her at ease.
- To allow for sound/vision problems:
  - Ask the patient to let you know if they are unable to hear or see you.
  - To test for sound delay: count "one, two, three" and have the patient count back immediately. Remember to pause for this amount of delay before responding in conversation.
- Have your EMR open for documentation in real time.
  - Two monitors or computers are ideal, but require high bandwidth.
- Use the "share your screen" option to share pictures and instructions.
- A chat window is very helpful (to send links, files, etc.).
- Send the patient after-visit instructions via secure, encrypted email (within electronic medical record if available) or mail.
- During times of uncertainty (e.g., COVID-19), follow-up may be challenging. Recommend providing the patient with a care plan several steps ahead, in case of uncertainty about the next follow-up.
- Send the patient's local medical care provider a letter or copy of your office notes, as for an in-office visit.
- Text chatting during the visit can be helpful. You can give simple instructions, write out difficult words (e.g., the diagnosis), provide web links, etc. Many video apps allow simultaneous texting as well. You can also consider separate text options.

Conclusions

The accelerated and profound changes in 2020 affecting how we deliver care to PD and movement disorder patients have been truly unprecedented.[19] Visual examination and description of movement disorders is traditionally and critically important in clinical practice and research (phenomenology) in this disease group. Considering the fact that most aspects of such visually rated examinations can readily be carried out in secure video conferencing assisted virtual visits, Parkinson's disease and movement disorders appear particularly well suited for teleneurology care conducted remotely. Added to that our growing reliance on objective motor measurements, such as motion sensors and other ecology valid tracking technology, referred to as "digital phenotyping",[12] it is easy to see why PD and movement disorders have played such a central role in the COVID-19 pandemic in the global adoption of teleneurology.[32,33] Teleneurology is already an inevitable part of how we care for PD and movement disorder patients, and while the COVID-19 pandemic has catalyzed teleneurology's adoption, it is evident that telemedicine delivery of care will permanently remain integral to how we care for patients with PD and movement disorder. There is hope that fiscal and regulatory changes prompted by the pandemic[13] will become permanent or even be expanded upon. I predict that the vast experience we have gained by relying on telemedicine during the pandemic will further catalyze the adoption of telehealth in PD and movement disorder practices by informing and guiding the regulatory, financial, and practice standards reforms beyond the pandemic.

References

1. AAN. *American Academy of Neurology Fellowship Directory*; 2020. https://www.aan.com/Fellowship.
2. Farbman ES. The case for subspecialization in neurology: movement disorders. *Front Neurol.* 2011;2:22.
3. MDS. *About Movement Disorders — by the International Parkinson and Movement Disorder Society*; 2020. https://www.movementdisorders.org/MDS/About/Movement-Disorder-Overviews.htm.
4. Shih LC, Tarsy D, Okun MS. The current state and needs of north American movement disorders fellowship programs. *Parkinsons Dis.* 2013;2013. https://doi.org/10.1155/2013/701426, 701426.
5. Goetz CG, McGhiey A. The movement disorder society and movement disorders: a modern history. *Mov Disord.* 2011;26(6):939–946.
6. Robakis D, Fahn S, Kestenbaum M. Essential tips for videotaping a movement disorders patient encounter. *Mov Disord Clin Pract.* 2015;2(4):365–368.
7. Beck CA, Beran DB, Biglan KM, et al. National randomized controlled trial of virtual house calls for Parkinson disease. *Neurology.* 2017;89(11):1152–1161.

8. Hanson RE, Truesdell M, Stebbins GT, Weathers AL, Goetz CG. Telemedicine vs office visits in a movement disorders clinic: comparative satisfaction of physicians and patients. *Mov Disord Clin Pract.* 2019;6(1):65–69.
9. Srinivasan R, Ben-Pazi H, Dekker M, et al. Telemedicine for hyperkinetic movement disorders. *Tremor Other Hyperkinet Mov (NY).* 2020;10. https://doi.org/10.7916/tohm. v0.698.
10. Tarolli CG, Zimmerman GA, Goldenthal S, et al. Video research visits for atypical parkinsonian syndromes among fox trial finder participants. *Neurol Clin Pract.* 2020;10(1):7–14.
11. Bull MT, Darwin K, Venkataraman V, et al. A pilot study of virtual visits in Huntington disease. *J Huntingtons Dis.* 2014;3(2):189–195.
12. Bhidayasiri R, Mari Z. Digital phenotyping in Parkinson's disease: empowering neurologists for measurement-based care. *Parkinsonism Relat Disord.* 2020;80:35–40.
13. Hassan A, Mari Z, Gatto EM, et al. Global survey on telemedicine utilization for movement disorders during the COVID-19 pandemic. *Mov Disord.* 2020;35(10):1701–1711.
14. Government U. *166 Cong. Rec. S2272 - CARES ACT;* 2020. https://www.govinfo.gov/ app/details/CREC-2020-05-06/CREC-2020-05-06-pt1-PgS2272.
15. Kostick K, Storch EA, Zuk P, et al. Strategies to mitigate impacts of the COVID-19 pandemic on patients treated with deep brain stimulation. *Brain Stimul.* 2020;13(6):1642–1643.
16. Miocinovic S, Ostrem JL, Okun MS, et al. Recommendations for deep brain stimulation device management during a pandemic. *J Parkinsons Dis.* 2020;10(3):903–910.
17. Fasano A, Antonini A, Katzenschlager R, et al. Management of Advanced Therapies in Parkinson's disease patients in times of humanitarian crisis: the COVID-19 experience. *Mov Disord Clin Pract.* 2020;7(4):361–372.
18. Helmich RC, Bloem BR. The impact of the COVID-19 pandemic on Parkinson's disease: hidden sorrows and emerging opportunities. *J Parkinsons Dis.* 2020;10(2):351–354.
19. Cubo E, Hassan A, Bloem BR, Mari Z, Group MD-TS. Implementation of telemedicine for urgent and ongoing healthcare for patients with Parkinson's disease during the COVID-19 pandemic: new expectations for the future. *J Parkinsons Dis.* 2020;10(3):911–913.
20. Papa SM, Brundin P, Fung VSC, et al. Impact of the COVID-19 pandemic on Parkinson's disease and movement disorders. *Mov Disord Clin Pract.* 2020;7(4):357–360.
21. Stoessl AJ, Bhatia KP, Merello M. Movement disorders in the world of COVID-19. *Mov Disord Clin Pract.* 2020;7(4):355–356.
22. Bloem BR, Dorsey ER, Okun MS. The coronavirus disease 2019 crisis as catalyst for telemedicine for chronic neurological disorders. *JAMA Neurol.* 2020;77(8):927–928.
23. Ben-Pazi H, Browne P, Chan P, et al. The promise of telemedicine for movement disorders: an interdisciplinary approach. *Curr Neurol Neurosci Rep.* 2018;18(5):26.
24. Schneider RB, Biglan KM. The promise of telemedicine for chronic neurological disorders: the example of Parkinson's disease. *Lancet Neurol.* 2017;16(7):541–551.
25. Abdolahi A, Scoglio N, Killoran A, Dorsey ER, Biglan KM. Potential reliability and validity of a modified version of the unified Parkinson's disease rating scale that could be administered remotely. *Parkinsonism Relat Disord.* 2013;19(2):218–221.
26. International Parkinson and Movement Disorder Society Telemedicine Study Group; 2020. https://www.movementdisorders.org/MDS/About/Committees-Other-Groups/MDS-Study-Groups/Telemedicine-Study-Group.htm.
27. Cubo E, Mari Z. *Telemedicine in Your Movement Disorder Practice: A Step-By-Step Guide;* 2020. https://www.movementdisorders.org/MDS/About/Committees-Other-Groups/Telemedicine-in-Your-Movement-Disorders-Practice-A-Step-by-Step-Guide.htm.
28. Cubo E, Mari Z. *Telemedicine for Movement Disorders during the COVID-19 Crisis: How Does This Affect Us?* ; 2020. https://www.movementdisorders.org/MDS/Education/ Workshops-Conferences/MDS-Webinars/Telemedicine-for-Movement-Disorders-during-the-COVID-19-crisis-How-does-this-affect-us.htm.

29. *Global Review of Telehealth Regulations by Locale*; 2020. https://www.movementdisorders.org/telemed-faq.
30. Cohen BH, Busis NA, Ciccarelli L. Coding in the world of COVID-19: non-face-to-face evaluation and management care. *Continuum (Minneap Minn)*. 2020;26(3):785–798.
31. Bloem BR, Henderson EJ, Dorsey ER, et al. Integrated and patient-centred management of Parkinson's disease: a network model for reshaping chronic neurological care. *Lancet Neurol*. 2020;19(7):623–634.
32. Dorsey ER, Okun MS, Bloem BR. Care, convenience, comfort, confidentiality, and contagion: the 5 C's that will shape the future of telemedicine. *J Parkinsons Dis*. 2020;10(3):893–897.
33. Dorsey ER, Bloem BR, Okun MS. A new day: the role of telemedicine in reshaping care for persons with movement disorders. *Mov Disord*. 2020.

CHAPTER 8

Introduction to tele-psychology during the pandemic

Annette E. Brissett, PhD[a,b]

[a]Director of Psychological Services, Clinical Psychologist, Houston Psychology Consultants, Houston, TX, United States
[b]Director of Psychological Services, Clinical Psychologist, Brain Health Consultants and TMS Center, Houston, TX, United States

The COVID-19 pandemic has altered the way that health and mental health care is provided to the community, creating increased anxiety and fear of the unknown for many, disruption of regular daily activities of life, coping skills and social support, and necessitating social isolation for safety, and leading many to feel hopeless and helpless. However, it has also necessitated some useful changes in the practice and delivery of psychological services, allowing patients easier access to mental health services through the use of telehealth or remote platforms. Telehealth or telemental health is the delivery of mental health care services at a distance, using multiple technological communication means (internet, telephone, web-based video conferencing, etc.) to effectively assess and treat patients in need.

Prior to COVID-19, most states frowned upon the delivery of health/mental health care services via telehealth, seeing it as inferior to in-person care and fearing that technology might present challenges for the effective delivery of psychological services. In mid-March 2020, many state officials across the US quickly adapted to the immediate crisis created by COVID and the need many patients had to seek help. As a result, governors throughout the US adopted a more flexible approach to ensuring that patients' continuity of care would be maintained and began to view telemental health and telemedicine as an integral service that would ensure the safety of both patients and health providers, in light of a spreading COVID-19 virus with no effective treatment in sight. While most states were not fully equipped to manage the influx of need for telemental health delivery, they responded by being permissive of most telecommunications platforms that would allow patients to access care without disruption as a result of abrupt lockdowns and social distancing. Some state mental health associations offered immediate help via pro-bono services to those in remote areas or who would not otherwise have access to a mental health provider, allowing psychologists the opportunity to help, via telemental health, across the state despite financial or physical limitation.

Due to COVID, it became imperative that patients receive the same level of care virtually that they would in-office; there was initial skepticism as to whether telemental health would result in clinicians missing important visual or behavioral cues that could be seen in-office, or whether patients would feel comfortable using a phone, iPad, or other devices to seek help. Telemental health was launched, and one essential tool to ensure open communication about the process of telemental health was the use of patient consent for telemental health. Ensuring that patients were presented with the limitations of an online platform versus in-person treatment, as well as obtaining a patient's verbal consent and/or written signature prior to beginning telemental health treatment, helped to manage patient expectations. Consent for telemental health would address the limitations of technology that might cause interruptions or disconnections in treatment, as well as addressing the concerns of those who might feel that telemental health is less comprehensive than in-person methods for diagnosing certain disorders and, may result in inconveniences such as a need to return to in-office visits, or even breaches in privacy that may inadvertently occur in patient environments or otherwise if others gained access to networks during sessions. Some patients initially wondered if tele-therapy would feel impersonal as it involved limited face-to-face contact with their clinician. Most have expressed relief at the ease and convenience of having frequent access to great help.

When performing a telemental health visit, a host of information is important to ascertain. A thorough history is required including a current list of health conditions, prior diagnoses, prior treatments, a list of health providers, and medications. You will also need to gather contact information/living arrangements specifics and details of the patient's social support. By remotely gathering a comprehensive history, this allows the clinician to provide help to the client and the ability to collaborate with other providers should the need arise. Limitations may exist for those at high risk, and these individuals may not be suitable for a tele-therapy/tele-assessment modality. Those individuals who are at high risk may require more comprehensive screening and risk assessment, as well as safety plans that include local crisis resources and family support.

While obvious limitations exist in a telemental health approach as it relates to physical assessment, some self-report assessments may be scanned or sent electronically to the patient in advance; patients may also download certain assessments on patient portals. If some situations necessitate an in-person visit or assessment, extra precautions should be taken and pre-screening should be carried out so that both the patient and doctor remain safe. This would include face masks, UV light and fans, sterilizing surfaces, and testing materials after each patient is seen, maintaining adequate spacing in between patients and during in-office visits, and ensuring that the patient and psychologist are more than 6 ft apart in testing situations.

Many telehealth platforms existed prior to COVID-19, and others have emerged. Regardless of the remote platform chosen by the clinician, the key is to ensure familiarity with the technology, competency, and expertise, and to make sure that patients fully understand the process and technology in which they have agreed to participate. Many patients view telemental health as a positive resource, citing its convenience and ease of access to immediate expertise among its various benefits. Clinicians have also responded positively, stating that tele-therapy lowers cancellation rates, and allows psychologists the flexibility to reach more patients in rural or outer lying areas who are in need, reducing wait times and providing much-needed resources to meet patients' immediate needs. While the COVID-19 pandemic has caused most individuals to socially isolate and withdraw from normal routines as a matter of safety, it has also allowed for greater connection and access to professional expertise, right at one's fingertips, via tele-therapy. Though our world has surely changed as a result of the COVID 19 pandemic, it is encouraging to note that some practices, like telemental health, are here to stay and will forever positively change the landscape of mental health delivery.

CHAPTER 9

Tele-neuropsychology: Bringing neuropsychology into the future of health care delivery

Kenneth Podell, PhD[a,b]
[a]Director of Houston Methodist Concussion Center, Stanley H Appel Department of Neurology, Houston Methodist, Houston, TX, United States
[b]Associate Professor, Clinical Neurology, Weill-Cornell Medical School and Institute of Academic Medicine, Houston, TX, United States

Tele-technology has been around for a long time. The earliest use of tele-technology in the United States was smoke signals by Native Americans. The use of the telegraph and the invention of the telephone are all examples of tele-technology. The use of telehealth technology has steadily increased over the past several years.[1] However, the recent severe acute respiratory system corona virus-2 (SARS-CoV-2) pandemic hurdled telehealth technology to the forefront of health care delivery. In a matter of weeks after a national health care emergency was declared in the USA by the Department of Health and Human Services (HHS),[2] the delivery of health care was transformed under the Corona Virus Aid, Relief, and Economic Security Act (CARES Act) passed on March 20, 2020[3] by allowing telehealth technology to be used instead of the in-office visit without the typical restrictions and limitations that were in place for tele-technology pre-COVID-19.

Neuropsychology (NP) has been particularly transformed by televisits. NP testing requires an in-depth clinical interview and face-to-face administration of both paper-and-pencil and computerized tests. The CARES Act allowed for broad use of telehealth technology, including in-home NP testing. However, very few neuropsychologists were prepared for tele-neuropsychology (tele-NP).

Telehealth refers to all aspects of health and health care using tele-communication technology such as emails, faxes, telephone, computers data/information, electronic equipment, and wearable devices, and most commonly, at least for today's purpose, video interaction. Telemedicine specifically delivers health care to patients via telecommunication, and is defined as "the remote diagnosis and treatment of patients by means of telecommunication technology."[4] State law defines what constitutes telemedicine and telemedicine practice.

There are always advantages and disadvantages with the advent of any new technology, and telemedicine is no different.[5,6] Use and adaptation of technology was the most common roadblock to adopting tele-technology in a health care setting (11%), while resistance to change and cost (8% each) and age or ability of the patient to use tele-technology (5% each) were also hindrances. Table 9.1 highlights many of the advantages and disadvantages that we currently have in using tele-technology to deliver health care services. As the technology evolves and improves, advantages to using the technology will increase while the disadvantages decrease.

Our expertise as neuropsychologists brings more to the clinical evaluation than simply psychometric assessments.[7] In addition to (and sometimes in place of) psychometric assessments, we can use our multispecialty training to diagnose, educate, and treat or to create treatment plans through clinical interviews, record reviews, and qualitative aspects of neuropsychological assessments.[8] Such skills are particularly relevant and useful during the COVID-19 pandemic or when the clinical situation or population does not allow for formal neuropsychological test administration.

This chapter will review how tele-NP has evolved over time, with the critical research showing its reliability, feasibility, effectiveness and limitations; it will also address practical issues, billing, and ethical considerations, and offer tips for developing and improving your own tele-NP practice.

Table 9.1 Advantages and disadvantages of tele-neuropsychology.

Advantages	Disadvantages
• Accessibility—rural areas, transportation • Cost-effective • Ease of scheduling • Less anxiety for the patient	• Cost of and accessibility to technology • Unfamiliarity with technology • Control of testing environment • Nonverbal cues • Inability to see all the testing area

Patient satisfaction

Patient satisfaction is a key component for a successful telehealth program. Patients need to be confident in the delivery methods, technology, and perceived effectiveness. A 2017 meta-analysis showed that acceptance of change in health care delivery (in person vs. teleconferencing) is generational-based with older patients less likely to accept change, but there is a growing trend of older patients being more accepting of technology incorporated into health care.[9] However, what was striking was the resistance that health care providers initially experienced in using/accepting teleconferencing, with some doctors not wanting to adopt it. However, during a 5-year period in the mid-2010s, patients' expectations were met when using teleconferencing or a telephone. It also improved access for patients (from remote or far-away areas), communication with the provider, and outcomes for chronic illness. Similar findings were noted for tele-psychology (clinical) with good efficacy, outcome, and clinical response.[10,11] There does not appear to be any concerns for patient satisfaction in Spanish-speaking populations or Native American Indians.[12–14] It is highly likely that our current COVID-19 pandemic will only serve to increase patients' acceptance of the technology and improve patient satisfaction.

Issues such as reimbursement, regulatory limitations, technology, and ease of platform use prevented many doctors from using telemedicine pre-COVID-19 despite the known economic and access benefits to lower-income patients.[15] However, it has been conducive to certain areas of medicine such as radiology, psychiatry, and tele-stroke. As of 2016, health care providers' use of telehealth technology in the United States was very limited with only 15% of physicians used interactive teleconferencing (ranging from just under 10% to about 40%—emergency medicine).[16] Interestingly, that same survey showed that patients were more likely to use telehealth (about 20% more than doctors). It appeared that the size of the physician practice was a major factor in using teleconferencing, with only 8% of doctors doing so in practices with four or fewer physicians, compared to 25% of doctors in larger practices with more than 50 doctors. This changed after the Coronavirus Aid, Relief, and Economic Security Act (CARES) was passed, which allowed for ease of billing and reimbursement (and practicing across state jurisdiction) and likely acted as an incentive for doctors to use telehealth.

Research in tele-neuropsychology

Given the scope of this chapter, this section will be limited to videoconference-based tele-NP research. The use of the telephone to deliver focused auditory, verbal-based NP tests has been available since the 1980s—much longer than video-based tests—and has shown good applicability, reliability, validity, and ease of use.[17–20] Its obvious limitation is that only auditory, verbal-based tests (in terms of both administration and response) can be used.

Adults

In order to determine if tele-NP administration is equivalent to in-office face-to-face (FTF) administration, one needs to assess the same patients under both conditions relatively close together in time. Munro Cullum has led this research, which dates back to the early 2000s.[13,21–24] Brearly et al. performed a systematic review and meta-analysis addressing the effectiveness of tele-NP videoconferencing test administration compared to in-office FTF test scores.[25] A total of 12 studies were included in the meta-analysis ($n = 497$) looking at a wide range of healthy adults (aged between their 30s and their 80s) and those with diagnosed psychiatric and neurocognitive disorders. Results of the meta-analysis showed that untimed tele-NP tests allowing for repetition were only about 0.01 standard deviation (SD) different than the same tests administered FTF. Moreover, performance on verbally mediated tests such as Digit Span (DS) and list-learning paradigms were unaffected by videoconferencing administration. The sole exception was the Boston Naming Test, which typically showed − 0.1 SD. The authors opined that the standardized normative data for the verbally mediated tasks were applicable when the same tasks are administered via videoconferencing. They noted the challenges of administering motor tasks and found too much variability to interpret that data. The authors noted methodological variability between studies and recommended the establishment of tele-NP administration and service delivery standards.

In a more recent update, Marra et al.[26] had similar findings to Brearly et al.[25] but were able to look across ethnicity and countries. They found "strong support" for tele-NP administration of screening measures (Montreal Cognitive Assessment and Mini-Mental State Examination) and verbal-based tests such as language, list-learning, and attention/working

Table 9.2 Videoconferencing administration of neuropsychological tests with strong correlation with in-person administration for adults.[a]

Adults
- Hopkins Verbal Learning Test
- Verbal Fluency Test (both letter and category)
- Digit Span (both forward and backward)
- Boston Naming Test (15-item)
- Clock Drawing
- Neuropsychological Screening Measures
  - Mini Mental State Examination
  - Montreal Cognitive Assessment
  - Repeatable Battery for The Assessment of Neuropsychological Status

[a]Note: See Brearly et al.[25] and Marra et al.[26] for reviews.

memory tests (Boston Naming Test, Letter Fluency, Hopkins Verbal Learning Test, and Digit Span). Other measures were "promising" but lacked adequate research evidence. Table 9.2 provides a list of videoconferencing administered NP tests showing good feasibility, reliability, and validity compared to in-office testing.

A critical distinction between the above research and real-world tele-NP assessments is that the tele-NP research was done under controlled conditions: the subjects were brought into an exam room and completed the tele-NP assessment after it was set up by a technician in a controlled environment using high-quality, standardized equipment. The control of the environment and standardization of computer equipment (monitor, speakers, and mouse) and standardized presentation are factors under less control in a true home-based tele-NP assessment and can impact test scores that can lower scores based upon environmental factors and thus lead to misinterpretation of test scores (and invalidate the use of normative data based upon in-person administration). Few studies considered at-home tele-NP administration. This latter point is especially important and a critical weak link in the clinical utility and readily adopting home-based tele-NP at present.

The impact of cultural and language-related issues on tele-NP has not been systematically studied. However, two studies indicated that tele-NP can be successfully used in a Spanish-speaking population or in Native Americans living on a tribal reservation.[12–14]

Pediatrics

One can easily see the added difficulties of administrating neuropsychological tests remotely to a younger population with limited attentional spans,
ability to follow instructions, comprehension, and behavioral problems. Two
studies performed remote language, reading, and intellectual assessments
with good success and interrater reliability between the remote and the on-
the-ground clinician.[27,28] However, only one study systematically looked
at the comparability of scores between videoconference and FTF administration.[29] Using a pediatric multietiologic demyelinating clinical group,
Harder et al. administered the same battery of verbal-auditory, visual, and
visuo-motor-based neuropsychological tests via videoconference technology with the patient at home (the patient's parent helped with computer
setup but was not in the room during formal videoconference testing) and
FTF, counterbalanced across patients. Consistent with the adult literature,
scores across the two settings were highly consistent with high patient and
parent satisfaction ($\geq 90\%$).

In the Hader et al. study, subjects were likely less impaired than other
neurodevelopmentally compromised patients, thus allowing the patients to
take the tests without any assistance.[29] To that end, Pritchard et al.[30] described the considerations and specific challenges of rapidly adopting to pediatric tele-NP models, while Pederson et al.[31] presented a three-tier model
for tele-NP evaluations with neurodevelopmentally complex patients with
specific case examples and recommendations. The model consists of a clinical interview with a comprehensive neurobehavioral status examination.
This was used to determine if the model was enough to provide recommendations or if the patient was best suited for a "tele-screen" (additional
standardized parent- or self-rating scales and abbreviated intellectual measures), tele-testing, or required FTF testing.

Tele-NP models

There are three tele-NP models being used today: (1) at-home without an
examiner; (2) in-office with an examiner outside of the testing room; and
(3) remote testing with an examiner in the room. The at-home without an
examiner is the model that is of most interest to us in today's pandemic as
well as for future use, but also the one with the least amount of environmental control and poorer comparability to FTF testing and normative data
interpretation. The at-home model requires the patient to have adequate
computer hardware and connectivity, and a quiet environment. There are

risks of test and data security, and concerns about nonstandard test administration and the use of normative data collected in a standardized fashion. The in-office tele-NP is a "hybrid" model attempting to have better environmental control to ensure a more accurate and as close to standardized neuropsychological assessment as possible while maintaining physical distance. In this model, the patient physically comes into the office and into an exam room where a computer is set up for a tele-NP assessment while the examiner is in another room. The connection can be via internet or a closed-circuit television, which has better security. The neuropsychologist or psychometrician administering the tests has control over the testing environment (noise, distraction, test security, and prevention of any recording). Tests can be preorganized and placed in folders that the patient is instructed to use. This allows for using many visual-based and computerized tasks that are not readily available with an in-home assessment. Please note that in order to use computerized tests, the examiner will likely have to enter the room to set up the computer, adding a very minimal health risk. Under this model, at least during a health emergency, there is still increased risk of exposure to the patient. The third model uses a psychometrist "on the ground" administering neuropsychological tests to the patient in person. Obviously the psychometrist is well trained and has complete control over the environment, and a full standardized neuropsychological evaluation is possible. However, it is not suitable in an emergency such as the SARS-CoV-2 pandemic as it places the examiner (and even the patient) at a higher risk for contamination.

C. Munro Cullum has advocated using a "staging approach" for at-home tele-NP evaluations.[32,33] This staging approach requires you to determine if in-home tele-NP assessment will be viable before actually attempting it. The first stage requires a record review and sometimes a call to the patient and their family to determine if there is any evidence that at-home testing would not be possible. Examples include patients who do not have adequate computer hardware, do not have internet access, have difficulties seeing, or are older without a family member to assist in computer setup. Next, doing a videoconference clinical interview will help you determine the feasibility of having a successful tele-NP assessment. Look for how the patient interacts with the computer—do they have adequate cognitive abilities to follow directions? Does the patient have the correct computer setup (laptop or desktop computer, not tablet or cell phone)? Sufficient bandwidth, lighting, sound, and potential for distractions are all factors to consider. If you feel that the patient can successfully complete at-home test administration, then a date is arranged for the at-home tele-NP evaluation. Feedback is performed separately on a later date.

I have used the staged at-home model since the COVID-19 emergency was declared and a "psychometrist on the ground" model for the past 4 years remotely when caring for sports-related concussions. In a program sponsored by the Houston Texans and General Electric Corporation, I have evaluated and treated more than 200 high school student-athletes who sustained sports-related concussions, covering a 350-mile radius from Houston. I trained several certified athletic trainers in test administration and clinical examinations as I instruct and observe remotely. This often entails at least two or three visits and allows me to have detailed FTF feedback sessions with the student-athlete and parents.

"Connecting" with the patient

Establishing a therapeutic connection with the patient is critical in psychology. Nothing fully replaces being FTF with your patient and being able to read body language and other nonverbal cues. However, research shows that good patient rapport and clinical intervention are successful with virtual video visits in psychotherapy,[33,34] and that the majority of cognitively intact or impaired adults find tele-NP testing acceptable, with more than 90% being satisfied with tele-NP testing and almost 66% having no preference between traditional in-office or FTF testing.[29,35] Context often shapes a patient's satisfaction. In the current pandemic environment, consumer satisfaction with, and preference for, tele-NP should be higher than that reported 7 years ago, as more and more patients are trying to avoid excessive community contact. One can only anticipate better acceptance of tele-technology as it becomes more integrated into health care delivery.

Improving clinical outcomes

Tele-NP testing can improve diagnosis and clinical outcomes for patients who otherwise would not have access to clinical services because of travel/distance or transportation, for example. Harrell et al. showed that tele-NP assessments for elderly individuals living in remote areas (mean age 75; range 55–90 years old and living 100–180 miles from the clinic) improved clinical care by clarifying or correcting the clinical diagnosis in 87% of the elderly patients referred.[36] Moreover, additional comorbid psychological and psychiatric diagnosis were made in 62% of the patients seen for a tele-NP evaluation, allowing for additional treatment recommendations and improved outcomes. Barton et al. performed neurologic and neuropsychological testing with elderly veterans referred for memory complaints who lived far from the San Francisco Veteran's Administration Hospital.[37] The researchers were able to help with clinical diagnoses and treatment recommendations for the primary care doctors at another VA hospital who referred the patients. It appears that diagnoses and treatment recommendations made via tele-NP are valid and consistent with those made in FTF settings, at least for dementia in a geriatric setting.[38,39]

Improving tele-NP visits

Performing tele-NP visits is challenging under the best of circumstances. However, there are several things one can do to improve the quality of these visits. Table 9.3 provides a list of practical suggestions designed to improve the quality of your tele-NP visits. Always remember that it will take practice, and that you will run into glitches along the way. One cannot expect that tele-NP visits will go as smoothly as your in-office visits, and you need to accept that they will fail on occasion. Having an alternative plan will help in the long run. It is hoped that the visits will improve with technological advancements. There are a few published guidelines for conducting tele-NP visits. Two of them are older and pre-COVID,[40,41] while two were written specific for tele-NP evaluations during COVID-19.[8,26]

Connecting with the patient during teleconferencing is essential in improving the quality of the tele-NP evaluation. As in FTF neuropsychological evaluations, introducing yourself and starting with a little small talk helps relax the patient and ease them into the tele-NP visit. Explaining everything in detail about the visit is crucial to helping the patient, and anyone else who is involved in the visit, to understand what to expect and to be more relaxed.

Consent form

The consent form used for a tele-NP evaluation differs from your in-office consent form in that it must address issues specific to the videoconference aspect of the evaluation that are not pertinent to FTF evaluations. The American Psychological Association[42] and the Inter Organizational Practice Committee (IOPC)[8] have published useful outlines for what a videoconference consent form for a psychology and neuropsychology-based evaluation

Table 9.3 Tips for improving in-home tele-NP visits.

Preparing for the Tele-NP Visit

1. Ensure signed consent specific for the tele-NP visit is supplied.
2. Have a backup plan in case the video connection is lost. This can be as simple as using the telephone, but this will alter any testing you might have considered. Alternatively, it may require rescheduling. In either case, it is important to discuss the plan ahead of time.
3. Have an emergency plan in place. It is crucial for clinical care to have a plan or plans in place that can handle a variety of emergencies when you are not physically present. Clearly you need to have an emergency contact, but do you have to make sure that the emergency contact is available during your tele-NP? How will you handle a situation where the patient becomes suicidal or homicidal, or if the patient has a medical emergency, for example?

The Patient

1. Have prepared written instructions for the patient/family to follow for computer requirements, setting up software, and tips for setting up the home environment, information about the nature of the visit, and detailed emphasis of the importance of minimizing distractions and of test security.
   a. Remember that a full-sized computer screen (14″ or larger) is likely to be needed to ensure that the patient can see test material if visual-based. A cell phone will not work.
2. Consider a test run with the patient/family prior to the initial session.
   a. This can be delegated to a staff member to do when the appointment is made or at another time.

Formal Testing Session

1. Check the patient's lighting. This should come from in front of the patient and not behind or overhead. The patient might have to turn off overhead or background lights and close window blinds to improve the image quality for the clinician/examiner.
2. Adjust the patient's distance from the camera, if possible, to allow you to see more of the patient as needed.
3. Confirm that the patient's hardware is adequate.
4. Listen for any distracting environmental noise.
5. Check ability of the patient to hear instructions. You can use simple yes/no questions or commands.
6. Consider screening for visual acuity and auditory comprehension to ensure comprehension of materials. Simple visual matching or naming and simple auditory comprehension tests can be used. Do not use actual test stimuli for practice. The patient might have to increase the volume on their computer.
7. Confirm the patient's identity, location, backup plan, and emergency contact information.

The Clinician

1. Practice. As with any new skill or technique, practice helps work out glitches and mistakes and helps to improve efficiency and quality.
   a. Operating the software. Practice using the software so when you have your tele-visit you are familiar with operating the software and the visit will go smoothly.
   b. Sound quality. Background sounds seem amplified via teleconferencing. It is important to do a test run to see what it sounds like from the patient's side, working on achieving sound that is as normal as possible. Speaking slightly slower helps with enunciation and ensures clarity for the patient. Increase your level of physical animation but do not let your hands be in front of your face if you use a lot of hand gestures.
   c. Test administration. Make sure the stimuli are clear and accurate from the test-taker's view.

2. Camera. The camera should be at or close to face level, not overly above or below one's face. It is important to invest in a high-quality camera. Adjust the distance from the camera to try to give yourself a more realistic size from the patient's view.

3. Lighting. This should come from in front of your monitor and not from behind you. Ensure no windows are behind you when doing videoconferencing.

4. Background. Make sure the background is simple. A busy background can be distracting to the patient. **Do not** use the animated background images offered by some videoconferencing software or your own. These are often glitchy and distracting. Consider a plain room partition behind you.

5. Facial animation. Exaggerate your level of facial expression. This helps with establishing good rapport and communication with the patient.

6. Speech. Speak louder and slightly slower than usual to make sure the patient can clearly understand.

7. Look into the camera and not at the patient's image on your screen. This helps you connect with the patient as they feel you are looking directly at them.
   a. This may be hard to remember as you will want to see the patient's image often. Try moving the patient's image to be closer to your camera's lens, to minimize any shifting of the head or eyes.

8. Keep your hands below your face when talking.

or treatment should look like. Addressing the potential breach of confidentiality inherent in tele-communication is a main difference in a tele-NP consent form. The difficult part is being able to explain this in a practical manner. While you can cite the *potential* risk, one cannot give a more definitive or concrete explanation such as a percentage. However, you can state that the software being used is Health Insurance Portability and Accountability Act-compliant and that it is considered a "secure" connection.

Three other important components of a tele-NP consent form address distractions, the emergency plan, and test material/answer security. You need to impress upon the patient and any other individual involved in the tele-NP visit(s) the importance of zero distractions, and review with them potential sources of distractions (phone, pets in the house, others entering the room, loud noises from others in the home, etc.). It is imperative that the patient and other individuals involved in the evaluation fully understand and comply with the requirement not to record the evaluation and not to keep any test responses. You can explain that this is critical to maintain the integrity and sensitivity of the tests. To this end, have them turn off cell phones in your presence. However, you must be explicit in stating that you may electronically record some of their responses (for example, clocking drawing) but explain that the material is saved on a secure network or drive. In addition, ensure that the patient destroys any of the written material once it is saved securely. The third important component of the tele-NP specific consent form is the emergency plan. This must be explained and discussed in detail, given that the patient is not physically with you and you have less control over the environment. Being able to handle a potential suicidal patient or a medical emergency that arises during the tele-NP visit will take some effort and planning on the practitioner's part.

Neuropsychological reports

While the literature clearly shows that tele-NP can yield a reliable and accurate assessment with specific tests, there are limitations and deviations from a standard neuropsychological evaluation. These must be clearly addressed and noted in your written report to help explain and educate the reader on how the evaluation was conducted and describe any limitations or variances in administration, normative data, and thus interpretation.[8]

The IOPC recommends clearly stating in your report that tests were administered via videoconferencing (or telephone), and indicating which telehealth platform was used and how any test administration was modified or adapted for videoconferencing/telephone in a nonstandard manner.

The IOPC also explicitly suggests stating that interpretation was non-standard and how any differences in test administration might have impacted interpretation. The following is an example given by the IOPC recommendations:

> *Due to circumstances that prevent in-person clinical visits, this assessment was conducted using telehealth methods (including remote audiovisual presentation of test instructions and test stimuli, and remote observation of performance via audiovisual technologies). The standard administration of these procedures involves in-person, face-to-face methods. The impact of applying non-standard administration methods has been evaluated only in part by scientific research. While every effort was made to simulate standard assessment practices, the diagnostic conclusions and recommendations for treatment provided in this report are being advanced with these reservations.*
>
> **Bilder and Reise [8, p. 8]**

Billing tele-NP

Two major roadblocks to using tele-NP pre-COVID-19 were restrictions on the use of the technology clinically and billing. Medicare allowed for tele-psychology to rural areas under certain limitations, but at least temporarily, under the CARES Act, tele-NP is acceptable to use and bill for all patients. Details on billing tele-NP is regional and carrier-specific, so one must always confirm the details with the patient's health insurance carrier. The Center for Medicare Services has helpful information about billing telehealth services under Medicare (see "Resources" later in this chapter).

Health care in general, and neuropsychology specifically, have complicated and cumbersome billing technicalities during normal daily operations. Tele-technology adds an additional layer of complication. However, some of those limitations were removed with the CARES Act. Drs. Neil Pliskin, Gillaspy, and Puente created guidelines for tele-NP billing codes and reimbursement.[43] As of September 1, 2020, all neuropsychology (and psychology) Current Procedural Terminology (CPT) codes were reimbursable as televisits at the same rate as in-office testing. However, remember that while the Centers for Medicare and Medicaid Services (CMS), Aetna, Blue Cross/Shield, Cigna, United Healthcare, and Humana reimburse for telehealth in general, policies vary (see IOPC for state-by-state information on tele-NP reimbursement).[44] In addition, you should determine if your state has reimbursement parity for telehealth services, as only a handful have payment parity laws.[45]

There are two differences to note when submitting the charges. First, place of service (POS) must be "02" for the televisit rather than the standard

"011," which represents an out-patient office. All CPT codes billed for telehealth must include the "95" modifier ("synchronous telemedicine service rendered via a real-time interactive audio and video telecommunications system") to distinguish their mode of administration, given that the neuropsychological CPT codes are by default in-office face-to-face.

Interstate practice

Interstate compacts (ICs) are voluntary, multistate cooperatives that maintain state sovereignty and avoid federal oversight or intervention, allowing states to work cooperatively in many different areas.[46] ICs are legally binding with a self-regulatory system of operations functioning within federal regulations. Since states maintain sovereignty, the IC does not create a single set of guidelines or regulations. Instead, members of different states function or operate using the patient's state regulations. Interstate compacts have become more common (since World War II) with each state, on average, belonging to 25 ICs. Driving is an example of an IC. While each state regulates their citizens' licenses, all states allow you to drive in their state with another state license, but you must follow the rules and laws of the state you are driving in, with states reporting infractions back to the home state.

The Psychological Interjurisdictional Compact (PSYPACT) was made effective and functional in 2020. PSYPACT was created and is overseen by the Association of State and Provincial Psychology Boards (ASPPB). It was first approved in 2015 to "facilitate telehealth and temporary in-person, face-to-face practice of psychology across jurisdictional lines."[47] At the time of writing, there were 12 member states effective in PSYPACT with two states with enacted but not effective legislation and 12 more states with pending PSYPACT legislation.[48] The regulations for temporary in-state practice is different. See https://psypact.site-ym.com/ for details and procedures for licensing.[49]

Clearly the value of an IC for tele-psychology practice can have a significant impact on access for patients and the number of potential clients for the clinician. However, several factors can influence one's decision to practice interstate tele-psychology. First, issues of reimbursement, at both national and state levels, will be tricky. There is interest at the federal level for making telehealth care permanent. The extent and scope of this has yet to be determined or even debated, even though bipartisan bills have been introduced in Congress to make telehealth care permanent. In addition, the clinician must know the state laws in which the patient resides and you must be familiar with the area to make sure you can respond if an emergency arises during the evaluation or treatment of the patient. PSYPACT is in its infancy and if several factors fall into place, interstate tele-psychology may have a foothold in growing our field and improving access to individuals who typically are unable to access the psychological (and neuropsychological) care they need, and present clinical opportunities for psychologists.

Future of tele-NP

Neuropsychology in general is at a crossroads in health care. In order to be able to assist patients and the health care community, we must transform and adopt our assessment techniques to be more relevant to every growing and evolving technology in medicine.[8,50,51] Tele-NP is very much in its infancy[8] with several hurdles and stumbling blocks to overcome. To optimize tele-NP, we must be innovative in designing technology and neuropsychological tools specifically designed for tele-technology rather than retrofitting our current in-office tests onto our existing tele-technology. Tele-NP research (at least for videoconferencing) has been around for more than 25 years, yet very few practitioners used it pre-COVID-19, and did so without developing proper tests specific to the tele-NP environment. Granted, this has largely been fueled by the lack of reimbursement for tele-NP services before the COVID-19 pandemic. However, it appears that this has the potential to change for tele-NP, with CMS recommending the permanent expansion of telemedicine and Congress introducing a bipartisan bill that makes such changes permanent and CMS making dozens of tele-health services permanent in the 2021 fee schedule. https://www.cms.gov/newsroom/press-releases/trump-administration-finalizes-permanent-expansion-medicare-telehealth-services-and-improved-payment. While we do not know how third-party insurers will reimburse for telemedicine delivery, they typical follow the lead of CMS and there is growing interest in making tele-visits permanent after the CARES Act expires. https://www.ama-assn.org/practice-management/digital/after-covid-19-250-billion-care-could-shift-telehealth.

This is clearly an opportunity for those of us in the field of neuropsychology to adopt our assessment and intervention techniques to the ever-changing and evolving health care landscape. If we plan to stay relevant in health care we must, as a clinical practice, be transformative, creating neuropsychological assessment and intervention techniques that are well suited for videoconferencing.[8,51] This will be challenging and likely take years to develop fully. However, we must start now. Granted, development of computer technology and equipment that is available to the masses is a critical component, as it is with any aspect of telehealth care. Here are some suggestions to help get us there:

1. Research. There are two components to this. For the present, we need to have research looking at how to adopt current tests and address in-home assessment feasibility, reliability, and validity. This will help us transition to developing novel measures specifically designed for tele-NP.

2. Work with test developers. Many of our current neuropsychological measures can easily be adopted for video display and thus easily be used in tele-NP. However, none of the large developers and distributors of NP tests allow for this currently. Of course, issues of test security must be addressed, but likely are not insurmountable challenges. We need to work with the distributors of neuropsychological tests in making many of our current tests suitable for tele-NP and then develop novel tests specific for the tele-NP platform.

3. Education. There are two prongs to education in tele-NP. The first is educating current licensed neuropsychologists on the benefits, value, and limitations of tele-NP, and how to incorporate it into their clinical practice. The second is introducing tele-NP practice into our graduate programs. The best way to ensure the future of tele-NP, as well as of the field of neuropsychology, is to educate our future neuropsychologists.

4. Collaboration. The future of neuropsychology relies upon its ability to collaborate with other scientific fields, just as in other health care fields such as radiology and cardiology. Working with computer science engineers, for example, can help us develop the future tele-NP tools we so desperately need.

Resources

Below are a few resources pertaining to tele-NP. The list is not exhaustive and was compiled on August 26, 2020.

1. General
   a. American Psychological Association (APA): https://www.apa.org/topics/covid-19/index#telementalhealth
   b. National Academy of Neuropsychology: https://nanonline.org/nan/Professional_Resources/Telehealth_Resources/NAN/_ProfessionalResources/Telehealth_Resources.aspx
   c. International Neuropsychological Society: https://www.the-ins.org/

    d. Sports Neuropsychology Society: http://www.sportsneuropsychol-ogysociety.com/resources-and-publications

    e. Inter Organizational Practice Committee: https://iopc.online/teleneuropsychology

2. Billing/Reimbursement

    a. Medicare Billing for telehealth services: https://www.cms.gov/Outreach-and-Education/Medicare-Learning-Network-MLN/MLNProducts/Downloads/TelehealthSrvcsfctsht.pdf

    b. IOPC: https://iopc.online/teleneuropsychology-reimbursement

3. Insurance Coverage

    a. IOPC: https://iopc.online/state-by-state-teleneuropsychology-resources

Summary

The current state of tele-NP is in its infancy without formal standard of care or practice guidelines to follow. Clearly, there are guidelines set up by national organizations (APA, ASPPB, and IOPC) for practicing during the pandemic health care emergency, but none have proposed long-term procedures for everyday use of tele-NP. To survive and stay current, neuropsychology as a profession must make more effort and place more emphasis on doing the needed research to develop the formal guidelines and best clinical practice recommendations for tele-NP. The future of tele-NP must start now, and our relevance in health care will require us to develop, improve, and adopt tele-NP into our everyday practice. It will not replace our in-office visits, but it seems clear that the future of out-patient care (or at least a large portion of it) will require adopting tele-NP that is valid and relevant, which requires ingenuity and research in test development, administration, and normative data ensuring test security, validity, and ease of use. This chapter reviewed the current data supporting the use of tele-NP, billing, technology, and resources, and provided recommendations and tips to improve televisits and recommendations for the future.

References

1. American Hospital Association. *February 2019 Fact Sheet: Telehealth*; 2019. https://www.phe.gov/emergency/news/healthactions/phe/Pages/2019-nCoV.aspx. Accessed 25 August 2020.
2. U.S. Department of Health and Human Services. *Determination that a Public Health Emergency Exists*; 2020. https://www.phe.gov/emergency/news/healthactions/phe/Pages/2019-nCoV.aspx. Accessed 28 August 2020.

3. *Congress.Gov. H.R. 748 – Coronavirus Aid, Relief, and Economic Security Act or the CARES Act*; 2020. https://www.congress.gov/bill/116th-congress/house-bill/748. Accessed 28 August 2020.

4. *Oxford Dictionary*. Telemedicine; 2020. https://www.lexico.com/en/definition/telemedicine. Accessed 28 August 2020.

5. Kruse CS, Krowski N, Rodriguez B, Tran L, Vela J, Brooks M. Telehealth and patient satisfaction: a systematic review and narrative analysis. *BMJ Open*. 2017;7. https://doi.org/10.1136/bmjopen-2017-016242, e016242.

6. Wade SL, Raj SP, Moscato EL, Narad ME. Clinician perspectives delivering telehealth interventions to children/families impacted by pediatric traumatic brain injury. *Rehabil Psychol*. 2019;64(3):298–306.

7. Braun M, Tupper D, Kaufmann P, et al. Neuropsychological assessment: a valuable tool in the diagnosis and management of neurological, neurodevelopmental, medical, and psychiatric disorders. *Cogn Behav Neurol*. 2011;24(3):107–114. https://doi.org/10.1097/WNN.0b013e3182351289.

8. Bilder RM, Reise SP. Neuropsychological tests of the future: how do we get there from here? *Clin Neuropsychol*. 2019;33(2):220–245. https://doi.org/10.1080/13854046.2018.1521993.

9. Kruse CS, Karem P, Shifflett K, Vegi L, Ravi K, Brooks M. Evaluating barriers to adopting telemedicine worldwide: a systematic review. *J Telemed Telecare*. 2018;24(1):4–12. https://doi.org/10.1177/1357633X16674087.

10. Bolton AJ, Dorstyn DS. Telepsychology for posttraumatic stress disorder: a systematic review. *J Telemed Telecare*. 2015;21(5):254–267.

11. Varker T, Brand RM, Ward J, Terhaag S, Phelps A. Efficacy of synchronous telepsychology interventions for people with anxiety, depression, posttraumatic stress disorder, and adjustment disorder: a rapid evidence assessment. *Psychol Serv*. 2019;16(4):621–635. https://doi.org/10.1037/ser0000239.

12. Vahia IV, Ng B, Camacho A, et al. Telepsychiatry for neurocognitive testing in older rural Latino adults. *Am J Geriatr Psychiatry*. 2015;23:666–670.

13. Wadsworth HE, Dhima K, Womack KB, et al. Validity of teleneuorpsychological assessment in older patients with cognitive disorders. *Arch Clin Neuropsychol*. 2018;33:1040–1045.

14. Weiner MF, Rossetti HC, Harrah K. Videoconference diagnosis and management of Choctaw Indian dementia patients. *Alzheimers Dement*. 2011;7:562–566.

15. Savani S, Muzammil M, Saleh K, Muqueet A, Zaidi F, Shaikh T. Addressing cost and time barriers in chronic disease management through telemedicine: an exploratory research in select low- and middle-income countries. *Ther Adv Chronic Dis*. 2019;10. https://doi.org/10.1177/2040622319891587, 2040622319891587.

16. Kane C, Gillis K. The use of telemedicine by physicians: still the exception rather than the rule. *Health Aff*. 2018;37(12):1923–1930. https://doi.org/10.1377/hlthaff.2018.05077.

17. Nesselroade JR, Pedersen NL, McClearn GE, Plomin R, Bergeman CS. Factorial and criterion validities of telephone-assessed cognitive ability measures. Age and gender comparisons in adult twins. *Res Aging*. 1988;10(2):220–234. https://doi.org/10.1177/0164027588102004.

18. Duff K, Beglinger LJ, Adams WH. Validation of the modified telephone interview for cognitive status in amnestic mild cognitive impairment and intact elders. *Alzheimer Dis Assoc Disord*. 2009;23(1):38–43.

19. Lachman ME, Agrigoroaei S, Tun PA, Weaver SL. Monitoring cognitive functioning: psychometric properties of the brief test of adult cognition by telephone. *Assessment*. 2014;21(4):404–417. https://doi.org/10.1177/1073191113508807.

20. Matchanova M, Babicz MA, Medina LD, et al. Latent structure of a brief clinical battery of neuropsychological tests administered in-home via telephone. *Arch Clin Neuropsychol*. 2020. https://doi.org/10.1093/arclin/acaa111, acaa111.

21. Cullum CM, Weiner MF, Gehrmann HR, Hynan LS. Feasibility of telecognitive assessment in dementia. *Assessment.* 2006;13:385–390. https://doi.org/10.1177/1073191106289065.
22. Cullum CM, Hynan LS, Grosch M, Parikh M, Weiner MF. Teleneuropsychology: evidence for video teleconference-based neuropsychological assessment. *J Int Neuropsychol Soc.* 2014;20:1–6. https://doi.org/10.1017/S1355617714000872.
23. Chapman JE, Cadilhac DA, Gardne B, Popnsford J, Bhalla R, Stolwyk RJ. Comparing face-to-face and videoconfernece completion of the Montreal Cognitive Assessment (MoCA) in community-based survivors of stroke. *J Telemed Telecare.* 2019. https://doi.org/10.1177/1357633X19890788, 1357633X19890788.
24. Galusha-Glasscock JM, Horton DK, Weiner MF, Cullum CM. Video teleconference administration of the repeatable battery for the assessment of neuropsychological status. *Arch Clin Neuropsychol.* 2016;31(1):8–11.
25. Brearly TW, Shura RD, Martindale SL, et al. Neuropsychological test administration by videoconference: a systematic review and meta-analysis. *Neuropsychol Rev.* 2017;27:174–186.
26. Marra DE, Hamlet KM, Bauer RM, Bowers D. Valdiity of teleneuropsychology for older adults in response to COVID-19: a systematic and critical review. *Clin Neuropsychol.* 2020;34:1411–1452. https://doi.org/10.1080/13854046.2020.1769192.
27. Hodge MA, Sutherland R, Jeng K, et al. Agreement between telehealth and face-to-face assessment of intellectual ability in children with specific learning disorder. *J Telemed Telecare.* 2019;25(7):431–437.
28. Sutherland R, Trembath D, Hodge MA, Rose V, Roberts J. Telehealth and autism: are telehealth language assessments reliable and feasible for children with autism? *Int J Lang Commun Disord.* 2019;54(2):281–291.
29. Harder L, Hernandez A, Hague C, et al. Home-based pediatric teleneuropsychology: a validation study. *Arch Clin Neuropsychol.* 2020;35(8):1266–1275.
30. Pritchard AE, Sweeney K, Salario CF, Jacobson LA. Pediatric neuropsychological evaluation via telehealth: novel models of care. *Clin Neuropsychol.* 2020;34(7-8):1367–1379. https://doi.org/10.1080/13854046.2020.1806359.
31. Peterson K, Ludwig NN, Tenzin JD. A case series illustrating the implementation of a novel tele-neuropsychology service model during COVID-19 for children with complex medical and neurodevelopmental conditions: a companion to Pritchard et al., 2020. *Clin Neuropsychol.* 2021;35:99–114. https://doi.org/10.1080/13854046.2020.1799075.
32. Podell K, Cullum CM. Teleneuropsychology: bringing neuropsychology into the future of healthcare delivery. In: *APA 2020 Annual Convention August 6, 2020;* 2020.
33. Hilty DM, Ferrer DC, Parish MB, Johnston B, Callahan EJ, Yellowlees PM. The effectiveness of telemental health: a 2013 review. *Telemed Health.* 2013;19(6):444–454. https://doi.org/10.1089/tmj.2013.0075.
34. Gros DF, Morland LA, Greene CJ, et al. Delivery of evidence-based psychotherapy via video telehealth. *J Psychopathol Behav Assess.* 2013;35(4):506–521. https://doi.org/10.1007/s10862-013-9363-4.
35. Parikh M, Grosch MC, Graham LL, et al. Consumer acceptability of brief videoconference-based neuropsychological assessment in older individuals with and without cognitive impairment. *Clin Neuropsychol.* 2013;27(5):808–817. https://doi.org/10.1080/13854046.2013.791723 [Epub 2013 Apr 22].
36. Harrell KM, Wilkins SS, Connor MK, Chodosh J. Telemedicine and the evaluation of cognitive impairment: the additive value of neuropsychological assessment. *J Am Med Dir Assoc.* 2014;15(8):600–6006. https://doi.org/10.1016/j.jamda.2014.04.015.
37. Barton C, Morris R, Rothlind J, Yaffe K. Videotelemedicine in a memory disorders clinic: evaluation and management of rural elders with cognitive impairment. *Telemed J E Health.* 2011;17:789–793.

38. Martin-Khan M, Flicker L, Wootton R, et al. The diagnostic accuracy of telegeriatrics for the diagnosis of dementia via video conferencing. *J Am Med Dir Assoc.* 2012;13:8. https://doi.org/10.1016/j.jamda.2012.03.004.
39. Shores MM, Ryan-Dykes P, Williams RM, et al. Identifying undiagnosed dementia in residential care veterans: comparing telemedicine to in person clinical examination. *Int J Geriatr Psychiatry.* 2004;19:101–108.
40. Grosch MC, Gottlieb MC, Cullum CM. Initial practice recommendations for tele-neuropsychology. *Clin Neuropsychol.* 2011;25(7):1119–1133. https://doi.org/10.1080/13854046.2011.609840.
41. Joint Task Force for the Development of Telepsychology Guidelines for Psychologists. Guidelines for the practice of telepsychology. *Am Psychol.* 2013;68(9):791–800. https://doi.org/10.1037/a0035001.
42. APA; 2020. https://www.apa.org/practice/programs/dmhi/research-information/informed-consent-checklist. Accessed 28 August 2020.
43. *Inter Organizational Practice Committee Teleneuropsychology-Reimbursement.* https://iopc.online/teleneuropsychology-reimbursement;. Accessed 28 August 2020.
44. *Inter Organizational Practice Committee – state-by-state-teleneuropsychology-resources.* https://iopc.online/state-by-state-teleneuropsychology-resources;. Accessed 28 August 2020.
45. *APA 2019 Winter Newsletter.* https://www.apaservices.org/practice/good-practice/2019-winter.pdf. Accessed 28 August 2020.
46. *Council of State Governments – National Compacts.* https://www.gsgp.org/media/1313/understanding_interstate_compacts-csgncic.pdf. Accessed 28 August 2020.
47. *Psychology Interjurisdictional Compact.* https://www.asppb.net/page/PSYPACT. Accessed 28 August 2020.
48. *PsychPACT Map.* https://psypact.org/page/psypactmap.
49. *PsychPACT.* https://psypact.org/. Accessed 28 August 2020.
50. Casaletto KB, Heaton RK. Neuropsychological assessment: past and future. *J Int Neuropsychol Soc.* 2017;23(9–10):778–790.
51. Bott NT, Madero EN, Glenn JM, et al. Device-embedded cameras for eye tracking-based cognitive assessment: implications for Teleneuropsychology. *Telemed J E Health.* 2020;26(4):477–481. https://doi.org/10.1089/tmj.2019.0039.

CHAPTER 10

Sleep telemedicine

Pablo R. Castillo, MD

Program Director Sleep Fellowship, Neurology, Mayo Clinic, Jacksonville, FL, United States

Overview

In part due to the limited access and capability of sleep centers, the field of sleep neurology is in a suitable position for real-time, interactive, audio-video telecommunications (telemedicine). The American Academy of Sleep Medicine's (AASM) Taskforce on Sleep Telemedicine supports telemedicine as a means of advancing patient health, by improving access to the expertise of Board-Certified Sleep Medicine Specialists.

From the use of sleep home monitoring devices to PAP therapy data, technology provides an opportunity to reach sleep patients at their home where they feel safe (specially children or vulnerable adults), as opposed to their traveling to a sleep center.

The American Academy of Sleep Medicine (AASM) provides an implementation guide that suggested two models: Center to Home (C2H) or Center to Center (C2C). The C2H model uses the patient's own technology (laptop, smartphone, etc.) from wherever they choose to access remotely the sleep specialist. In the C2C model, the patient goes to a nearby location, typically a medical office or clinic where the equipment is located, and is then connected with a sleep specialist. Whatever model is available, having a private telecommunications channel that meets the technical requirements is a requisite (see Table 10.1).

Sleep telemedicine diagnostic approaches

Sleep is affected by circadian rhythms, light, backgrounds, sleep patterns, and other environmental variables. The zeitgeber action of light is influenced by interaction between circadian and homeostatic processes, and the opportunity to assess the home sleep environment is valuable to enhance the sleep interview. Nocturnal Artificial Light exposure (NLE) can be harmful by activating the melanopsin system in the retina, which will result in melatonin suppression. NLE can be assessed by asking the patient to show the amount

Table 10.1 Technical provisions for sleep telemedicine.

Bandwidth: Minimum connection speed @ 384 kbps; videoconferencing software.

Resolution: Minimum live video services @ 640×480 resolution at 30 frames/second.

Software: Software and operating system should be up to date with the latest security updates.

Diagnostic equipment: Electronic stethoscope and additional peripheral devices are encouraged to be used if they can aid clinical needs.

Safety: Compatible with published regulations for devices used in patient care and infection control procedures followed.

Privacy: Use of encryption for both live and stored information, inactivity timeout function, protected health information, and confidential data only stored on secure data storage. Access granted only to authorized users.

Adapted from AASM Position Paper for the Use of Telemedicine. Singh J, Badr MS, Diebert W, et al. American Academy of Sleep Medicine (AASM) position paper for the use of telemedicine for the diagnosis and treatment of sleep disorders. J Clin Sleep Med. 2015;11(10):1187–1198. doi:10.5664/jcsm.5098.

of luminosity generated by their light bulbs. This can be determined by reading the manufacturer's package, and also by the use of devices that measure luminous intensity or brightness (luxometers); these are also available as smartphone applications. One hundred lumens is equivalent to about 20 watts, and at higher levels, melatonin alterations can be expected. (It should be noted that most interior designers, unaware of the impact of light on sleep and circadian rhythm, recommend up to 2000 lm for a bedroom.) Measures to decrease NLE further include reducing the light intensity of smartphones, TVs, and computers by activating their nighttime modes, and the use of lenses that filter harmful blue light.

Bedroom temperature verification is simply done by inquiring about thermostat temperature settings at night (see Table 10.2).

Table 10.2 Factors influencing the sleep environment.

1. Nocturnal artificial light exposure.
2. Nocturnal utilization of electronic devices
3. Bedroom temperature verification.
4. Mattress with signs of wear and tear.
5. Environmental noises.
6. Partner discord
7. Potential for injury.

Tips when taking a sleep history and performing the sleep-oriented exam

Conducting a sleep history via telemedicine should be performed according to the same professional and clinical care standards expected during face-to-face office visits. At the time of this publication, there are no completed trials assessing the noninferiority of the management of neurological sleep disorders (new diagnosis or established diagnosis) such as restless legs syndrome, parasomnia, and narcolepsy via telemedicine compared to usual in-office care.

Most of the sleep exam, including airway inspection and measurement of neck size (using the neck grasp technique, or a measuring tape), can be carried out via telemedicine. An examination assisted by external or intra-oral cameras can be conducted to phenotype the upper airway. With optimal light and zoom view, testing of palate elevation and tongue movements can be achieved.

A general setup for airway video examination of the oral airway includes the following:

1. A well-lit room, avoiding sources of light behind the patient's head. Ideally, patients should be sitting on a chair. Use an additional light source to enhance visualization of oropharynx subsites (tonsils, etc.).
2. Have a second person nearby to assist in tasks.
3. The chin and neck should also be visible, in order to look for bumps or masses.
4. Examine the back of the patient's mouth by asking them to use a spoon as a tongue depressor.

In certain situations, the sleep physician may demonstrate the optimal examination technique on themselves first. In this way, patients may learn not to obstruct the physician's view when doing it themselves.

1. **Obstructive Sleep Apnea (OSA):** There are several validated surveys that can be use via telemedicine to identify individuals at risk for sleep apnea. The most commonly used are the STOP-Bang and Berlin questionnaires; administration of these requires approximately 8 min and 2 min to complete, respectively.
2. **Insomnia:** The assessment of insomnia severity can be easily achieved by using the insomnia severity index, a 7-item Likert-type scale, which takes about 5 min for completion with total scores ranging from 0 to 28. Cognitive behavioral therapy for insomnia (CBT-I) can also be conducted via telemedicine, by addressing the thoughts and behaviors that promote insomnia.

3. **Narcolepsy:** The sleep neurologist should ask about primary symptoms of narcolepsy including excessive daytime sleepiness, sleep-related hallucinations, sleep paralysis, and sudden loss in muscle tone triggered by mostly positive emotions (cataplexy), which is not to be confused with exaggerated startle response. Excessive daytime somnolence can be formally assessed by administering validated tools including the Stanford Sleepiness Scale and/or the Epworth Sleepiness Scale.

4. **Parasomnias:** Safety is a major component of parasomnia management. A safety assessment can be done by a video walk-through of the patient's sleeping environment, and observing the bedroom area for potentially injurious obstacles such as furniture or glass windows.

Additionally, visiting the bedroom facilitates better recall of the nocturnal motor activities, including answers to two important questions: "Does the patient wander outside the bedroom during the event?" and "Does the patient perform complex directed behaviors?"

Before asking the patient to perform certain tasks, it is important to have an assistant or caregiver at home, in order to prevent falls during examination. The use of automatic speech recognition captioning can assist telemedicine evaluations dealing with patients who have clinically significant hearing loss.

A unique benefit of televisits performed in the patient's home is the ability to examine their sleep environment. The sleep neurologist can request the patient to demonstrate their ability to change positions in bed and the ability to transfer in and out of bed. The presence of orthopnea can also be noted in the supine position, which may suggest neuromuscular weakness. Careful observation may allow optimization of position restriction therapies, by observing the use of mechanical devices to avoid supine sleep.

Bedroom evaluation may be helpful to identify elements that may affect sleep quality. While validation is still needed, the use of a structured exploration of the sleep environment may help identify predisposing and precipitating factors that may contribute to circadian rhythm alterations, sleep disruptions, and insomnia. Table 10.1 shows factors to include in a structured questionnaire for assessment of the sleep environment.

Safety assessment of the sleep home environment related to both the patient and the sleeping partner is particularly revealing via telemedicine. When dealing with cases of potentially injurious parasomnias (such as rapid eye movement (REM) sleep behavior disorder or agitated sleep walking), observation of adequate positioning of barriers on the side of the bed/

padding the floor near the bed and removal of sharp items, weapons, sharp edges furniture, glass windows, and clutter from the bed area are crucial to prevent injuries.

Sleep diagnostics and interpretation of sleep studies should be in accordance with the AASM Manual for the Scoring of Sleep and Associated Events. The use of home sleep studies, other than polysomnography (PSG), is now a widespread standard of care. Home-based PSG recordings include electroencephalogram (EEG), electrooculogram (EOG), and electromyogram (EMG), and requires appropriate bandwidth with data transfer to a virtual cloud-based platform for sleep scoring and archiving of raw data (see Table 10.1).

Sleep telemedicine treatment approaches

In order to effectively manage sleep apnea patients remotely, wireless positive airway pressure (PAP) transmission of therapy data is essential. Home PAP devices have modems that enable them to send data to the manufacturer's server (cloud-based platform), which can be accessed by the medical equipment company, patient, and sleep specialist.

Real-time titration of auto PAP has been available for some time, and there is ongoing continued development in technology including long-term home polysomnography, with remote positive airway pressure titration.[1,2]

Other telemedicine sleep treatment applications include treatment for insomnia. In a randomized noninferiority trial, telemedicine delivery of cognitive behavioral therapy (CBT) for insomnia was not inferior to face-to-face encounters for insomnia, with similar improvements on daytime functioning outcomes.[3]

The AASM taskforce endorses the use of live interactive telemedicine as an alternative for prescription of sedative hypnotics, stimulant medications, wakefulness-promoting medications, or other controlled substances prescribed by the sleep specialist.

Telemedicine follow-up approaches

The cloud-based platform becomes a source of a large amount of data which can help promote engagement of patients by access to education resources, efficacy of treatment (residual apnea-hypopnea index), adherence, assessment of mask leaks, and troubleshooting of common problems. Active patient engagement using technology is beneficial in terms of improving daily PAP use; however, the use of these applications may inadvertently exclude less technically savvy patients.[4] Nevertheless, evidence suggests that adherence to PAP is improved with telemedicine.[5]

Smartphone applications, smartwatches, and even finger rings are widely distributed among consumers Those applications are multiple and use technologies including movement sensor, microphone, video, oximetry, actigraphy, and ballistocardiography to measure sleep stages, although validation data are lacking.[6]

Another aspect that is likely to interact with telemedicine is the ever-changing use of consumer sleep technologies (CSTs). Sleep apps remain among the most popular apps downloaded for smartphone devices, and their utilization continues to increase. The lack of validation data and absence of Food and Drug Administration (FDA) clearance raise concerns about the accuracy of CST data. CST tools are not substitutes for formal sleep evaluation; however, as long as sleep neurologists acknowledge CST-gathered sleep data, CSTs may enhance clinical interaction by improving patient engagement.

Furthermore, the tracking of objective data using CSTs, with the resultant self-correlation with daytime function, may lead to an unrealistic and anxious pursuit for the perfect sleep. This condition has been named orthosomnia.[7]

Additionally, therapies other than PAP, including dental devices, have the potential to be monitored remotely using thermal sensors implanted into the dental device by reading the device at mouth temperature vs. room temperature (device taken out of the mouth).[8]

Conclusion

Sleep telemedicine offers a unique opportunity for the enhancement of clinical data pertaining to the sleep history and the home sleep environment. Widespread application of sleep telemedicine should maintain ethical and clinical care standards expected in face-to-face office visits.

Sleep telemedicine is a fast-moving scenario with potential concerns of limited compensation. Progress of financial regulations and protocols in telemedicine is required to sustain further implementation by patients and sleep specialists.

References

1. Dellaca R, Montserrat JM, Govoni L, et al. Telemetric CPAP titration at home in patients with sleep apnea-hypopnea syndrome. *Sleep Med*. 2011;12:153–157.
2. Kristo DA, Eliasson AH, Poropatich RK, et al. Telemedicine in the sleep laboratory: feasibility and economic advantages of polysomnograms transferred online. *Telemed J E Health*. 2001;7:219–224.
3. Arnedt JT, Conroy DA, Mooney A, Furgal A, Sen A, Eisenberg D. Telemedicine versus face-to-face delivery of cognitive behavioral therapy for insomnia: a randomized controlled non-inferiority trial. *Sleep*. 2020;44(1). https://doi.org/10.1093/sleep/zsaa136, zsaa136.
4. Malhotra A, Crocker ME, Willes L, Kelly C, Lynch S, Benjafield AV. Patient engagement using new technology to improve adherence to positive airway pressure therapy: a retrospective analysis. *Chest*. 2018;153(4):843–850. https://doi.org/10.1016/j.chest.2017.11.005.
5. Fox N, Hirsch-Allen AJ, Goodfellow E, et al. The impact of a telemedicine monitoring system on positive airway pressure adherence in patients with obstructive sleep apnea: a randomized controlled trial. *Sleep*. 2012;35(4):477–481. https://doi.org/10.5665/sleep.1728.
6. Jaworski DJ, Roshan YM, Tae CG, Park EJ. Detection of sleep and wake states based on the combined use of actigraphy and ballistocardiography. *Conf Proc IEEE Eng Med Biol Soc*. 2019;2019:6701–6704. https://doi.org/10.1109/EMBC.2019.8857650.
7. Baron KG, Abbott S, Jao N, Manalo N, Mullen R. Orthosomnia: are some patients taking the quantified self too far? *J Clin Sleep Med*. 2017;13(2):351–354.
8. Vanderveken OM, Dieltjens M, Wouters K, De Backer WA, Van de Heyning PH, Braem MJ. Objective measurement of compliance during oral appliance therapy for sleep-disordered breathing. *Thorax*. 2013;68(1):91–96. https://doi.org/10.1136/thoraxjnl-2012-201900.

CHAPTER 11

Neuromuscular evaluation

Ericka Greene, MD[a,b]

[a]Associate Professor, Education Director of Neurology, Division Head, Neuromuscular Medicine Houston Methodist Neurological Institute, Houston, TX, United States
[b]Curriculum Director, Practice of Medicine, EnMed, Texas A&M University College of Medicine, College of Engineering, Houston, TX, United States

The history of telemedicine

Telemedicine is the remote diagnosis and treatment of patients by means of telecommunications technology.[1] However, this simple definition does not reflect the history of its development, which has been integrated with technology, and innovation. Like many technological advances that are now common to our daily lives and professions, telemedicine was birthed alongside the birth and growth of the internet in the 1960s. One of its earliest uses in medicine was the use of the satellite 'Early Bird' which allowed Dr Michael Debakey to conduct an aortic valve replacement while engaging with surgeons in the Director-General of the WHO and other surgeons in Geneva Switzerland.[2] Fast forward to 2020, and the marriage of the internet and technology has created a diverse and broad telecommunication platform accessible not only to governments, world organizations, and institutions, but also to civilians, from the clinician and systems-based providers to the individual health care consumer.

Telemedicine in neurology

However, it was the use of telemedicine in stroke care that actually paved the way for the application of telemedicine in neurology practice settings. Telestroke services have been an essential part of acute stroke care for more than a decade, integrated with improved access, quality of care, and treatment rates with evidence of equitable outcomes.[3] Until recently, with the advent of the COVID-19 pandemic, the advances witnessed with telestroke services have been limited in use for other neurological conditions.

Prior to the COVID-19 pandemic and its impact on society, and more specifically the delivery of quality health care, discussion of telemedicine use in neurology was limited to a minority of ambulatory practices with great variability in how it was used among clinicians and their practices. Most publications discussed the potential of telemedicine across different subspecialties and approaches to delivery, from multidisciplinary care clinics to rural isolated practices. Most publications reported noninferiority of telemedicine evaluations to in-person evaluations in regards to disease outcomes as well as patient and clinician satisfaction related to increased access, decreased travel, and costs per visit. Yet there has been minimal evidence showing utility across various settings and cultures, and even less evidence regarding its impact upon clinical outcomes in large cohorts,[3] including that of neuromuscular medicine.

Telemedicine in neuromuscular disease

Neuromuscular conditions include a wide range of disorders with a broad range of etiopathogeneses, diagnostics approaches, and treatments. Some are rare, listed among the rare orphan diseases, such as amyotrophic lateral sclerosis. Others are more common, such as diabetic polyneuropathy. Thus, the approach to the diagnosis and management of these conditions also varies in terms of the types of care settings where neuromuscular patients receive care.

Telemedicine in ALS

Amyotrophic lateral sclerosis is a diagnosis of exclusion requiring a detailed examination and thorough testing. In addition, the disease requires a comprehensive multidisciplinary approach, typically at a tertiary center or practice with such an affiliation. In contrast, diabetic polyneuropathy and headache patients are managed across a variety of clinical care settings (urban, rural, academic, private), by generalists and specialists alike. Similar to other subspecialties, there is a paucity of randomized, blinded studies of telemedicine in neuromuscular medicine, with small, less robust studies focusing on patient and caregiver perception and satisfaction.[4]

Neuromuscular disorders like ALS require subspecialized care, in-depth history and examination, interdisciplinary care, and extensive assessments and testing. These disorders also present special challenges in accessing health care due to impairments in mobility and function. This is further complicated in that the majority care is provided at tertiary medical centers with up to 25% of patients (e.g., ALS) living more than 100 miles away from such centers.[4] Nonetheless, although there has been limited experience utilizing telemedicine for neuromuscular disorders across practice settings, there are reported benefits to its use in this patient population.

Amyotrophic lateral sclerosis is a neurodegenerative disorder of predominant motor neurons resulting in progressive motor disability of limbs and bulbar and respiratory functions. ALS patients benefit from the care of multidisciplinary care teams in terms of quality of life and survival,[5] making the disease amenable to telemedicine in order to address the needs of the patient who is unable to access health care consistently in person (distance and disability). The application of telemedicine in ALS attempts to bridge the gap in care for such patients, who are often lost to follow-up, or transition their care to single provider clinics or home health agencies that provide physician or physician equivalent care.

One of the two applications of telehealth is by direct clinical video teleconferencing with the ALS care team. Van De Rijn et al.[6] conducted a retrospective review of 136 videos for nearly 100 ALS patients living 10–3136 miles from the care center. The team provided televisits to both ambulating patients (> 50%) as well as more advanced patients on invasive ventilation (23%) and those receiving home hospice care (11%). Although limited by the retrospective design, notable benefits included convenience for patients at all stages of disease, extension of care to more advanced patients, and opportunities to engage other care providers in the encounter who otherwise might not have attended an in-person visit. Limitations identified include variability in the adoption of technology among patients and even providers, as well inconsistency of reimbursement at the time of the study.[6]

In terms of outcomes, most reported no difference in disease progression for patients evaluated at regular intervals via televisits compared to patients seen in-person.[7] Most reported high patient acceptance and satisfaction of telehealth services, only preferring in-person visits for psychosocial issues that may require in depth disclosure.[8,9]

Another application of telehealth for ALS patients is the monitoring of ventilator compliance to manage parameters and use by accessing stored data from a data chip uploaded to a central site.

These interventions are associated with decreased emergency room visits and admissions. Similarly, a review of these studies found an overall benefit associated with decreased time and cost of travel by patients and increased patient satisfaction,[6] as well as better management of palliative care.

Despite the benefits of telemedicine in the care of ALS patients, obvious challenges and questions remain as to its use and implementation in providing multidisciplinary care for this population. Logistical issues exist regarding assembling a team of providers for the encounter, as well as for the patient, who may not have resources or ability to access the technology. Furthermore, the vulnerability of the platform to technical difficulties, both external (e.g., weather) or internal (system support disruptions) remain as variables that are difficult to control.

Care centers have taken a variety of approaches to address this issue. Some have provided telecare that is primarily led by the physician or physician extender, who triages the patient needs or issues to team members who evaluate the patient at a separate time, either virtually, telephone or video, or in person if indicated. Prior to the COVID-19 pandemic of 2020, others used telehealth in combination with a home visit program in which the physician/physician extender remained remote and teleconferenced with team members who assessed the patient at their home. This latter approach addresses the limitation of performing a virtual examination as well as ensuring the accuracy and standardization of assessment and measures of disease for clinical care and research.

In 2019, Pulley et al. reported on the *store and forward method* for multidisciplinary ALS care, in which a patient is assessed by a trained provider, such as a nurse, at the patient's home. The assessment is recorded and reviewed by individual team providers who send their recommendations to the clinic director within a week of the home visit. These recommendations are communicated to the patient by the clinical director via videoconferencing, or telephone communication, with the nurse present during a second home visit. The authors reported uniform patient satisfaction, although there was some variable response by providers regarding time to report recommendations and satisfaction with depending upon a proxy evaluator. This approach allowed patients to remain at home, including those who would otherwise be lost to follow-up due to advanced disease. However, in addition to limited to no reimbursement for team members, the authors noted challenges with managing the storage of large data files and quality of data capturing, as well as variable provider satisfaction with technology.[10]

Another approach is to incorporate telemedicine encounters with in-person multidisciplinary clinics, thus allowing the homebound and those living significant distances away, the opportunity to be evaluated by the team of providers. This approach has been shown effective both before the restrictions of the pandemic[8] and in response to the pandemic, with many providers across specialties providing care via a hybrid of in-person and telemedicine encounters within a multidisciplinary clinic.

It is also important to acknowledge that the use of telemedicine in the multidisciplinary care of neuromuscular patients is not restricted to a model that is solely focused on the neurologist as the primary provider. Telemedicine can also provide patients access to subspecialized therapy services including pulmonary and respiratory services, neurorehabilitation, assistive technology, and durable medical equipment evaluation, as well as neuropsychology, caregiver support, and palliative care.

In reference to home monitoring of non-invasive positive pressure ventilation and invasive ventilation, telemedicine has provided an avenue for providers to acquire measures of respiratory function and oxygenation that are incorporated into pulmonary rehabilitation, which was first documented in lung transplant patients in the 1990s.

Neurorehabilitation and home safety evaluations via telemedicine provide continuity of care for neuromuscular patients who would otherwise require serial visits. This was first pioneered by the Veterans Health Administration and has been associated with improvements in mobility, cognition, and quality of life, with superior results on functional outcomes compared to standard care.[11,12] These benefits have also been seen with customized seating for wheelchair via telehealth wheelchair seating clinics.[4]

Cognitive screening and complete neuropsychological assessments have been performed and are associated with improvements in coping skills, mood, and quality of life, especially when combined with behavioral therapy and patient support and networking. Similar benefits have been reported with programs that address caregiver wellness, although these studies were not specific to caregivers of neuromuscular patients.

Telemedicine in ALS and neuromuscular disorders clearly addresses issues related to patient access, cost, and burden associated with in-person care. It also provides opportunities for remote monitoring and management of related functions of respiration, rehabilitation, cognition, and well-being. Patient satisfaction is consistently rated as high among patients and providers, with some relative variability among the latter. Limitations include the lack of an examination, variability in technology access and support, as well as the ever-moving target of reimbursement, and state-specific limitations of practice.[4]

Despite an increasing number of studies of the use of telemedicine in neurology and neuromuscular disorders, the breadth of studies in neuromuscular medicine lack sufficient methodology to evaluate robustly its impact on disease outcomes including mortality, function, quality of care, cost, and the impact on emergent evaluation of the acute patient.

Further research is indicated but is challenged by issues related to blinding of patients and providers to the intervention, inherent selection bias for patients who can access and navigate the platform, as well as the lack of standardization of care and outcome measures across diseases and practice settings. Furthermore, such studies need expansion to other chronic neuromuscular disorders, which would likely benefit from improved access, subspecialized care, and improved outcomes. Just as important is the need to examine the role of telehealth for those disorders with a more subacute or fluctuating clinical course, such as myasthenia gravis, and its impact on outcomes of costs, functional outcomes, quality of life, and satisfaction.

Telemedicine in neurology in the COVID-19 era

As the COVID-19 pandemic impacted the globe and the Unites States, the focus of health care centered on managing acute cases of COVID-19 in the setting of strained resources and health care providers, with an upswing in investigations of established and experimental therapies. With restrictions of social distancing and imposed isolation, a significant gap was created in providing care for ambulatory patients, and the provision of elective surgical and nonsurgical assessments and interventions. This gap required a rapid increase in telehealth applications across the broad spectrum of practices and settings due to the COVID-19 emergency. As a direct result, telemedicine visits increased by 50-98% across institutions and specialties.[13,14]

Rapid transition to telehealth required expansion of coverage by federally supported and private payers, a temporary loosening of restrictions under the Health Insurance Portability and Accountability Act, expansion of physician licensing across state lines, and a rapid expansion of telehealth capacity. These measures allowed the ramp-up needed to provide care for patients for continuity of care, to address and triage emergent issues, and to provide a sense of support during an unsettling time.

The pandemic created a steep learning curve for neurologists whose knowledge of telemedicine was limited to its application in acute stroke care and a small number of academic and private settings. In a few months, neurologist learned to navigate existing platforms and technology and translate the components of the history and examination from a face-to-face encounter to a virtual encounter.

The speed and efficiency by which practitioners were able to make this transition was dependent upon the specialty and practice setting, as well as the presence of an existing telemedicine platform, and the bandwidth of the technology and that of its users.

The field of neurology includes an increasing number of subspecialties, which cover a subset of disorders and assessments that differ in reliance upon the examination or procedural assessments and treatments. Therefore, for subspecialties in which the history is central to the encounter, the transition to telemedicine actually provided a seamless path for providing continuity of care. This has been the experience for epileptologists, for whom the remote monitoring and assessment of seizures was already established for most practices. In epilepsy, both patient and providers have experienced benefits from the ease of scheduling follow-up encounters for ongoing patient issues without the burden of travel from home.[15] Telemedicine for these patients seems to work well when paired with existing remote electrophysiologic monitoring, although it may not be adequate for new patient evaluation.

Telemedicine in neuromuscular medicine in the COVID-19 era

In neuromuscular medicine, transitioning to telemedicine was associated with unexpected benefits for both practitioner and patient, as well as challenges. Some shared by all of neurology, and some unique to the specialty.

Similar to previously published reports prior to COVID-19, our patients report high satisfaction with telemedicine due to it enabling safe sheltering, and involving less burden and cost associated with travel for face-to-face encounters. Visualization allowed patients to demonstrate their home environment as well as issues related to medical devices. Furthermore, family members and caregivers were able to participate in the encounter and assist with assessments if needed. Physician satisfaction was based on the ability to provide assessment from remote locations, providing continuity of care for those patients with relatively stable disease, nonemergent medicine adjustments, and triaging patients for additional testing or in-person assessments.

However, because assessments of a patient with neuromuscular disease often rely on a thorough history and examination, the telemedicine neuromuscular encounter has required clinicians to translate the neuromuscular examination virtually. While certain aspects of the exam can be assessed, albeit superficially, through visualization, other aspects of the exam (motor power, reflexes, fundoscopic, muscle tone) can not be performed virtually.[16]

Neurologists have had to adopt new approaches to acquiring examination information from their patients without prior training or certification, often focusing on examination components that are considered more objective, easily demonstrated or instructed to the patient, and clearly visualized (oculomotor function, muscle bulk, symmetry of movement, speech, coordination, mentation, speech/language).

During this COVID-19 era, neuromuscular specialists consider this less-than-optimal assessment acceptable in the context of a patient with relatively stable disease. However, for a newly referred neuromuscular patient or a patient with unstable or active clinical disease, the virtual neuromuscular examination cannot replace an in-depth neuromuscular in-person evaluation.

Reliance upon telehealth has required creative approaches to the televisit by both provider and patient. Similar to the in-person encounter, patients' bandwidth to prepare for the telehealth visit also varies. For some patients, comfort and competence with virtual technology remains a significant barrier to accessing telehealth. This has ranged from an inability to connect properly—reducing a visualized encounter to a limited telephone encounter—to a lack of "production" skill, with poor or misdirected placement of camera view or audio settings. In contrast, other patients may prepare for their telehealth visit well in advance, including ensuring proper connectivity and access, providing vitals via wearable or home devices, and ensuring proper positioning and visualization for adequate assessment. In addition, it is important to consider the impact of other social determinants of health, such as education, culture, race, and age, that historically have impacted access to care, also apply to telemedicine in both similar and novel ways.

The Virtual Examination of the Neuromuscular Patient

The approach to the virtual examination by neuromuscular specialists varies according to the patient and sub-specialty. Some specialists depend on straightforward visualization and observations that require little of the patient in terms of maneuvers (facial symmetry, speech, extraocular movements, and observed upper body range of motion), whereas other specialists may provide the patient with validated patient surveys for objective assessment or written and/or visual aids that provide instruction on the examination, or ask the patient to enlist a capable family member/spouse to assist with the examination (Video 11.1 on Expert Consult).

The incorporation of existing validated surveys and scales has provided objective assessments of function, disease progression, and symptom burden in neuromuscular medicine. Prior to COVID-19, use of these tools for diseases like amyotrophic lateral sclerosis (ALSFRS, CNS-Lability scale), myasthenia gravis (MG -ADL, MG QoL15), and neuropathy (VAS, INCAT) was limited to patients receiving care in specialized or multidisciplinary clinics involved in translational or clinical trial research. Although the current use of these tools in telemedicine for neuromuscular conditions has not been quantified, many of these measures have become an integral part of the telemedicine neuromuscular examination based on ease of administration by patients, caregivers, or providers. As practitioners continue to navigate delivery of care during the pandemic, it is likely that such tools and possible newly developed tools will become an integral part of the neuromuscular assessment across practice settings and neuromuscular disorders, including for respiratory function.[17]

Wilson et al.[18] constructed a neuropathy scale from 10 existing validated assessments (Fig. 11.1). The investigators measured concordance between the newly constructed Veterans Affairs Neuropathy Scale (VANS) with documentation of neuropathy status based on chart review as well as

The VA Neuropathy Scale

Romberg 0=normal 1=step off	Casual Gait 0=normal 1=abnormal	Heel Walk 0=normal 1=abnormal	Tandem Walk 0=normal 1=abnormal

Left Knee Reflex 0=normal or brisk 1=absent or depressed	Right Knee Reflex 0=normal or brisk 1=absent or depressed
Left Foot Inspection 0=normal 2=ulcers, skin fissures	Right Foot Inspection 0=normal 2=ulcers, skin fissures
Left Toe Vibration 0=normal 1=decreased 2=absent	Right Toe Vibration 0=normal 1=decreased 2=absent
Left Knee Vibration 0=normal 1=decreased 2=absent	Right Knee Vibration 0=normal 1=decreased 2=absent

Segments for pin sensation reporting

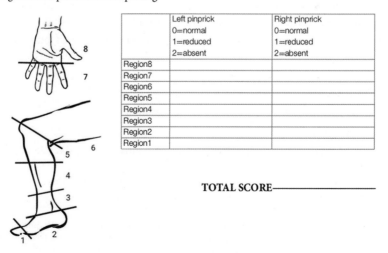

	Left pinprick 0=normal 1=reduced 2=absent	Right pinprick 0=normal 1=reduced 2=absent
Region8		
Region7		
Region6		
Region5		
Region4		
Region3		
Region2		
Region1		

TOTAL SCORE————————————

Fig. 11.1 The Veterans Affairs Neuropathy Scale (VANS).[18]

the reliability of results between in-person vs. remote grading by board-certified neurologist vs. nonneurologist evaluators (telemedicine technician, medical assistant, and nurse), respectively. The VANS incorporates assessment of neuropathy findings as well as those for balance, mobility, and skin integrity.

The VANS has a sensitivity and specificity of 98% and 91%, respectively, for identifying peripheral neuropathy and a correlation coefficient of 0.89 across scenarios of in-person or remote assessment and physician or nonphysician evaluator, although in-person assessments grades were higher than remote assessments independent of type of evaluator. This pilot study highlights the promise of such scales for remote assessments that demonstrates reliability between raters and correlation with in-person assessment. However, the authors concede that it may not detect milder disease with a lower pretest probability and does not replace the gold standard of an in-person assessment. It is also not clear from the study what is required of patients for training with assessments and their intra rater and inter rater reliability.[18]

Future progress in the development of valid and reliable tools that aid in remote assessment will need to show an acceptable concordance between the in-person and remote assessments. In addition, newly developed tools and surveys, will need to be administered easily by patient or caregiver, time efficient, comprehensive, and sensitive for meaningful use. Table 11.1 provides a list of patient-reported surveys and tools for disease progression, disability, or function, which can be easily incorporated into telehealth assessments for common neuromuscular disorders.

In the absence of a standardized approach to the virtual neurology examination, provision of guidelines and instructional resources presently lags behind the need, although there is an appreciable number of publications

Table 11.1 Disease-Specific Tools for Neuromuscular Assessment.

Neuromuscular disease	Assessment tool[a]
Myasthenia gravis	MG – ADL, MG–QoL 15
Chronic inflammatory demyelinating neuropathy	INCAT, inflammatory-RODS
Painful neuropathy	Visual analog scale, TNAS
Amyotrophic lateral sclerosis	ALSFRS, CNS-LS

[a]Myasthenia Gravis-Activities of Daily Living, Myasthenia Gravis Quality of Life 15, Inflammatory Neuropathy Cause and Treatment Disability Score, Inflammatory Rasch-built Overall Disability Scale, Treatment-induced Neuropathy Assessment Scale, Amyotrophic Lateral Sclerosis Functional rating scale, Center for Neurologic Study-Lability Scale.

addressing virtual assessment[16] as well as the landscape of biomedical technology that is being stretched to address the needs by both industry and federal parties.[19,20]

From our experience, the ability to perform a virtual neuromuscular examination successfully depends on many factors above and beyond the telehealth platform being used and access to IT support. At a minimum, it requires a certain technological and mental bandwidth of both clinician and patient. Another factor is the degree of preparation provided by the physician and patient to help to optimize the encounter. Preparation includes: (1) having the patient check for connectivity and bandwidth in advance of the visit; (2) performing a preassessment to determine what aspects of the examination require evaluation; (3) providing patient-reported assessments in advance that can be completed before or during the visit; and (4) providing direction regarding setting up device(s) for proper visualization of the patient and their surroundings. The clinician should also be prepared to demonstrate the required maneuvers to the patient during the visit, especially for the initial telehealth encounter. The participation of a willing and capable spouse or family member to assist with the examination can also provide valuable information as well as the incorporation of commercial or personal tools or devices for testing (e.g., sensory testing) (Table 11.2).

Table 11.2 The Virtual Examination of the Neuromuscular Patient.

Objective	Examination	Supplemented examination with assistant or device/tool
Cranial nerves	Pupils: Observe for symmetry then reaction to light by having the patient cover and uncover each eye independently.	Pupils: Use of light source in darkened room.
	Oculomotor function: Look in the nine cardinal positions of gaze with brief pause at each position. Sustained vertical gaze (60–120 s) by fixating on an object or ceiling.	Directing eye movements with finger or tool (pen, light source) in nine cardinal positions and for sustained (60–120 s) vertical gaze.
	Curtain sign: Ask patient to lift more ptotic eyelid and look for the less ptotic lid to become more ptotic.	Facial strength: resistance testing of jaw and oral and orbicularis muscles.

(Continued)

Table 11.2 The Virtual Examination of the Neuromuscular Patient—cont'd

Objective	Examination	Supplemented examination with assistant or device/tool
Motor	Facial strength: Ask patient to lift eyebrows, squeeze eyes shut, show teeth, and purse their lips, observing for any asymmetry.	
	Oral buccal/speech: Listen for dysarthria, dysphonia. Repetition of lingual, (l's) labial (p's), and guttural (k's) sounds.	Visualization of gag reflex and palatal elevation with light source.
	Tongue: Observe the tongue at rest for bulk and fasciculations, then ask patient to stick out tongue and move it side to side.	Other: palpation of head and neck.
	Assess muscle bulk in upper and lower limbs.	
	Observe for abnormal movements in the limbs. Assess for pronator drift and forearm rolling.	
	Neck flexion: Patient turns head right and left and then shrugs shoulders.	Resistance testing (≥ 4 out of 5) of neck flexion and extension, sternocleidomastoid, and trapezius muscles.
	Assessment of symmetric antigravity (3 out of 5) power, have the patient move through a full range of motion in both upper and lower limbs.	Resistance testing (≥ 4 out of 5) of muscles of upper and lower limbs (with safe positioning of patient).
	Extended elevation of arm at shoulder (120–240s) to test for fatigability.	
	Extension of leg at knee in the seated position or at hip in supine position (120–240s) to test for fatigability.	
	Ability to squat and rise to standing position.	Assistance as needed for safety.
	Rising from a seated position without use of arms.	Assistance as needed for safety.
	Ability to stand or walk on toes or heels.	Assistance as needed for safety.

Table 11.2 The Virtual Examination of the Neuromuscular Patient—cont'd

Objective	Examination	Supplemented examination with assistant or device/tool
Sensory	Ask the patient to compare light touch sensation (index finger) of face, arms, and legs.	Patient or assistant can use tools: Cotton tip or monofilament (light touch), end of opened paper clip (sharp), cooled or warmed utensil (temp.).
	Proximal to distal gradient testing for limbs and torso as indicated.	Position sense testing by assistant (may require demonstration and instruction). Vibration testing (patient or assistant) of distal/proximal joints if tuning fork or comparable device available.
Coordination/ tone	Visualization of rapid-alternating, finger-to-nose (or finger-to-object or screen), and heel-to-shin movements.	Assist with passive range of movement (ROM) of limbs to assess tone, rigidity, contractures.
Gait and balance	Observe stance and ability to stand with feet together.	Assistance as needed for safety.
	Observe gait, and ability to walk in tandem.	Assistance as needed for safety.
	Observe heel and toe walking.	Assistance as needed for safety.

Adapted and modified from Hussona MA, Maher M, Chan D, et al. The virtual neurologic exam: instructional videos and guidance for the COVID-19 era. Can J Neurol Sci 2020;47:598–603. https://doi.org/10.1017/cjn.2020.96.

Conclusion

Each clinician must choose an approach to teleneurology that best fits their patient population. Flexibility and creativity are needed to accommodate the evolution of the technology and the variable maneuverability of both clinician and patient. It is likely that the future of health care for neurology and associated subspecialties will be indelibly marked by a hybrid of in-person and remote assessments. As a consequence, standardized approaches to telehealth are expected to emerge soon in order to provide guidance for all stakeholders including federal and private payers, technology and industry partners, and institutions of medical education and accreditation (Videos 11.2–11.4 on Expert Consult).

References

1. Oxford Dictionary. *Lexico*; 2020. August 8. Retrieved from Lexico.com https://www. lexico.com/en/definition/telemedicine.
2. Doarn RC. Editorial: the journal, telemedicine, and the Internet. *Telemed e-Health*. 2014;293–295.
3. Hatcher-Martin JH, Adams JL, Anderson ER, et al. Telemedicine in neurology: telemedicine work group of the american academy of neurology. *Neurology*. 2020;94(1):30–36.
4. Howard IA. Telehealth applications for outpatients with neuromuscular or musculoskeletal disorders. *Muscle Nerve*. 2018;58:475–485.
5. Traynor BJ, Alexander M, Corr B, Frost E, Hardiman O. Effect of a multidiscplinary amyotrophic lateral sclerosis(ALS) clnic on ALS survival: a population based study, 1996–2000. *J Neurol Neurosurg Pyschiatry*. 2003;74:1258–1261.
6. Van De Rijn M, Paganoni S, Levine-Weinberg M, et al. Experience with telemedicine in a multi-disciplinary ALS clinic. *Amyotroph Lateral Scler Other Motor Neuron Disord*. 2018;19(1–2):143–149.
7. Selkirk SM, Washington MO, McClellan F, Flynn B, Seton JM, Strozewski R. Delivering tertiary centre specialty care to ALS patients via telemedicine: a retrospective cohort analysis. *Amyotroph Lateral Scler Frontotemporal Degener*. 2017;18(5–6):324–332.
8. Geronimo A, Wright C, Morris A, Walsh S, Snyder B, Simmons Z. Incorporation of telehealth into a multidisciplinary ALS clinic: feasibility and acceptability. *Amyotroph Lateral Scler Frontotemporal Degener*. 2017;18(7–8):555–561.
9. Nijeweme-d'Hollosy WO, Janssen EP, Huis in 't Veld RM, Spoelstra J, Vollenbroek-Hutten MM, Hermens HJ. Tele-treatment of patients with amyotrophic lateral sclerosis (ALS). *J Telemed Telecare*. 2006;12(Suppl 1):31–34.
10. Pulley MT, Brittain R, Hodges W, et al. Multidiscplinary amyotrophic lateral sclerosis telemedicine care: the store and forward method. *Muscle Nerve*. 2019;59:34–39.
11. Chumbler NR, Quigley P, Li X, et al. Effectts of telerehabilitation on physical function and disability for stroke patients: a randomized, controlled trial. *Stroke*. 2012;43:2168–2174.
12. Levy CE, Silverman E, Jia H, Geiss M, Omura D. Effects of physical thterapy delivery via home video telerehabilitation on functional and health-related quality of life outcomes. *J Rehabil Res Dev*. 2015;52:361–370.
13. Mouchtouris N, Lavergne P, Montenegro TS, et al. Telemedicine in neurosurgery: lessions learned and transformation of care during the COVID-19 pandemic. *World Neurosurg*. 2020;140:e387–e394.
14. Roy B, Nowak RJ, Roda R, et al. Teleneurology during the COVID-19 pandemic: a step forward in modernizing medical care. *J Neurol Serv*. 2020;414. https://doi. org/10.1016/j.jns.2020.116930, 116930.
15. Berlin J. The tele-future is now: will telemedicine's footprint be permanent post-COVID-19? *Tex Med*. 2020;116(7):14–19.
16. Hussona MA, Maher M, Chan D, et al. The virtual neurologic exam: instructional videos and guidance for the COVID-19 era. *Can J Neurol Sci*. 2020;47:598–603. https://doi. org/10.1017/cjn.2020.96.
17. Kukulka K, Gummi RR, Govindarajan R. A telephonic single breath count test for screnning of exacerbations of myasthenia gravis: a pilot study. *Muscle Nerve*. 2020;62:258–261.

18. Wilson AM, Ong MK, Saliba D, Jamal NI. The veterans affairs neuropathy scale: a reliable, remote polyneuropathy exam. *Front Neurol*. 2019;10. https://doi.org/10.3389/fneur.2019.01050, 1050.

19. FDA. *Digital Health*; 2020. August 27. Retrieved from fda.gov https://www.fda.gov/media/106331/download.

20. Leo S. *Living with New Realities: The Future Of Virtual Care*; 2020. July 6. Retrieved from Forbes Business Council: https://www.forbes.com/sites/forbesbusinesscouncil/2020/07/06/living-with-new-realities-the-future-of-virtual-care/#1cf17bd38c14.

CHAPTER 12

General neurosurgery exam

Jonathan J. Lee, MD, Gavin W. Britz, MD, MPH, MBA, FAANS
Department of Neurosurgery, Houston Methodist Hospital, Houston, TX, United States

Introduction

A thorough yet focused neurological examination of a patient has been the cornerstone of any neurosurgery clinician's training. Although the value of the human touch and in-person evaluation of a patient at the bedside or in a clinic setting cannot be understated, an effective neurosurgical examination can be performed via telemedicine, specifically by use of interactive video calls. In fact, many neurosurgeons were forced to convert many of their patient visits to virtual visits during the COVID-19 pandemic. During this time, instead of the doctor stepping from one clinic room to the next, neurosurgeons were taking live video calls through laptops or cell phones, interviewing and examining patients through screens. Additionally, in contrast to the vast majority of high-risk patients from outside hospitals being immediately transported to larger, more equipped hospitals, emergency room physicians were video calling on-call neurosurgeons while examining patients to determine if transfers to their far-away centers were fully warranted.

A focused neurosurgical interview via telecommunication takes a patient and inquisitive clinician. In Chapter 3, the reader learned the how to evaluate a stroke patient, the basics of which are similar to the general neurosurgical exam. In Chapters 5 and 6, the reader was introduced to the ophthalmological exam, which has many similar components to the eye component of the neurosurgical exam. In this chapter, the reader will be introduced to the basics of a general neurosurgical exam and how best to implement this exam in a remote setting.

Introductory interview questions

All patients should be asked the typical medical interview questions, such as past medical history and surgical history. Other pertinent history questions include chronic medications, such as blood thinners and antiepileptic medications, and family history of disease. All patients should also be asked about handedness (left- or right-handed). Handedness can give an accurate assessment of the laterality of language dominance in patients. One study found that the incidence of right-hemisphere language dominance was found to increase linearly with the degree of left-handedness, from 4% in strong right-handers, to 15% in ambidextrous individuals, and 27% in strong left-handers.[1]

Mental status

Alertness

To begin the general neurosurgical exam, the clinician must quickly assess the patient's alertness and appropriateness to introductory questions. If a patient is drowsy upon first inspection, this may be a sign of something pathological in the brain, such as hydrocephalus or an intracranial hematoma. If the patient is difficult to arouse, the best course of action should be to send this patient to an emergency department to obtain a noncontrasted head computed tomography (CT).

Orientation

After introducing yourself, there are three orientation questions that can assess if the patient is oriented appropriately:
1. "What is your full name?"
2. "Where are we?" or "What place are we in currently?"
3. "What is today's date?" or "What year and month is it today?"

These questions ask the orientation on three separate levels: person, place, and time. It is important to understand what the patient's baseline cognition is before these questions are asked. For instance, if a patient has diagnosed dementia, he or she may not answer these questions correctly at all in the first place. Additionally, if the patient has had a traumatic brain injury (TBI) in the past, his or her appropriateness to these questions may be disrupted on a regular day. The neurosurgical practice of reporting orientation is to say the patient is "oriented *times*" some numerical number out of three, which can be qualified immediately afterwards. For example, "Mrs. Jones was only oriented times 1—to person," or "The patient was oriented times 3." If the clinician is confident that the patient has a normal baseline, any disruption in orientation should raise suspicion.

Level of consciousness

The Glasgow Coma Scale (GCS) is a quantifiable tool used to assess a patient's level of consciousness and is widely used among neurosurgery clinicians worldwide. The GCS was originally devised in 1974 as a simple bedside tool to better communicate a patient's level of consciousness in a wide range of disorders.[2] Additionally, there has been strong evidence that the GCS correlates with clinical outcome in an extensive list of pathologic states, including TBI (see Table 12.1).[3-5]

The GCS ranges from a score of 3 to 15. The GCS is widely used scale to assess outcomes in TBI[6] and is used as a common classification of the severity of the injury:

- Severe, GCS 3–8;
- Moderate, GCS 9–12;
- Mild, GCS 13–15.

A score of ≤ 8 denotes that the patient is in a coma, although a full clinical picture needs to be taken into account. The historical teaching to emergency medicine practitioners was that any patient with a GCS ≤ 8 requires endotracheal intubation; however, many investigators and clinicians argue against this dogma.[7] There may be subtle, reasonable reasons why a person's GCS may be low that may not be directly related to an injury itself

Table 12.1 Glasgow coma scale.

Behavior	Response	Score
Eye opening	Spontaneous	4
	Response to verbal command	3
	Response to pain	2
	Eyes remain closed	1
Verbal response	Oriented	5
	Confused	4
	Inappropriate words	3
	Incomprehensible words	2
	No verbal response	1
Motor response	Obeys commands	6
	Localizes to pain	5
	Withdraws to pain	4
	Flexion to pain	3
	Extension to pain	2
	No motor response	1

(e.g., recent pain medication given). The authors use GCS mainly as a communication tool among other clinicians and use it to supplement the report of the neurologic exam.

Troubleshooting the GCS examination via telecommunication

For obvious reasons, the motor exam may be the most difficult component of the GCS exam to elicit over a video call. If the patient fails to obey commands to verbal cues, another practitioner would need to be present to perform the exam.

Speech

During the interview, speech and language should also be assessed by the examiner. Specifically, fluency, repetition, and naming are the most commonly examined components of speech to the neurosurgeon. These components can easily be assessed via remote telecommunication (see Table 12.2).

After knowing the patient's handedness (see above section on Introductory Interview Questions), it is possible to localize speech and language dysfunction to a specific hemisphere. Broca's and Wernicke's aphasia are two common aphasia syndromes.[8] Aphasia is a term used to describe a disturbance in the ability to use symbols (written or spoken) to communicate information.[9] It is important to distinguish aphasia from dysarthria, which is the inability to articulate speech secondary to a motor dysfunction (e.g., from CNs IX, X, or XII), but fluency and comprehension remain normal.

A Broca's aphasia, also known as expressive aphasia, is manifested as the partial or completely loss of the ability to produce language (spoken, manual, or written), although the patient retains the ability to comprehend

Table 12.2 Focused language examination.

Element	Description	Prompt
Fluency	Quantity, rate/rhythm	Fluency can be tested by having the patient speak conversationally. Assess for paraphasic errors.
Repetition	Repetition of phrases and words	Ask to repeat a common phrase, such as, "Today is a sunny day in Houston."
Naming	Naming objects	Show the patient three objects and ask him/her to say the name of the object aloud.

language. A Broca's aphasia is of particular interest to the practicing neurosurgery clinician because it is a localizing lesion—the most common cause of Broca's aphasia is a stroke involving the dominant inferior frontal lobe, usually of the middle cerebellar artery (MCA) or the internal carotid artery (ICA).[9] Other causes of a Broca's aphasia include TBI and mass occupying lesions, such as a tumor or abscess.

A Wernicke's aphasia, also known as receptive aphasia, manifests as the inability to comprehend language. Patients can have normal articulation, rate, and rhythm, which is why this aphasia is also known as having a "fluent aphasia." The most common cause of Wernicke's aphasia is an ischemic stroke of the posterior temporal lobe.[10]

Cranial nerve exam

The cranial nerve (CN) exam tests the 12 cranial nerves of the central nervous system. After the mental status components, this is typically the next component to be assessed in the general neurosurgical examination.

As can be seen in Table 12.3, all cranial nerves of a patient can be assessed remotely. It would be useful if another live examiner were with the patient on the other end of the virtual call. Generally, it is not necessary to test every component of each cranial nerve (e.g., parasympathetic actions of some). Nevertheless, if any dysfunction of a cranial nerve is observed on

Table 12.3 Cranial nerve examination.

Cranial nerve	Function	Remote exam maneuver
I (Olfactory)	Olfaction (sensory)	Have patient smell a strong odor (e.g., coffee).
II (Optic)	Vision (sensory)	Ask about changes in visual acuity. Have patient read from a written source. The examiner can also test visual fields.
III (Oculomotor)	Extraocular muscles, levator palpebrae muscle (motor); pupillary constriction, ciliary muscles (parasympathetic)	Ask patient to move eyes in all directions. Assess the patient's eyelids for ptosis. Ask examiner/patient to shine a light in both eyes.

(Continued)

Table 12.3 Cranial nerve examination—cont'd

Cranial nerve	Function	Remote exam maneuver
IV (Trochlear)	Extraocular muscle, superior oblique (motor)	Ask patient to move eyes in all directions.
V (Trigeminal)	Facial, corneal, nasal/oral cavity, anterior two-thirds of the tongue sensation; muscles of mastication, tensor tympani (motor)	Have examiner test facial sensation. Ask patients to produce a chewing motion.
VI (Abducens)	Extraocular muscle, lateral rectus (motor)	Ask patient to move eyes in all directions.
VII (Facial)	Taste of anterior two-thirds of tongue (sensory); facial expression, stapedius (motor); salivary and lacrimal glands (parasympathetic)	Ask patient to smile and keep eyes shut against resistance from live examiner.
VIII (Vestibulocochlear)	Hearing, vestibular system (sensory)	Have examiner or patient test finger rub in each ear.
IX (Glossopharyngeal)	Sensation and taste of posterior one-third of tongue, pharynx (sensory); stylopharyngeous muscle (motor); salivary glands (parasympathetic)	Ask patient to open mouth and say, "Ah."
X (Vagus)	Pharynx, larynx, thoracic and abdominal viscera (sensory); soft palate, pharynx, larynx (motor); multiple parasympathetic actions	Ask patient to open mouth and say, "Ah."
XI (Accessory)	Sternocleidomastoid, trapezius (motor)	Ask examiner or patient to turn chin against resistance of the contralateral face. Ask patient to raise both shoulders.
XII (Hypoglossal)	Tongue muscles (motor)	Ask patient to stick out tongue and move from side to side.

examination, the patient should be referred to an emergency department or a facility capable of performing an immediate noncontrasted head CT.

A special note on cranial nerve III and VI palsies

A more detailed explanation of the ophthalmologic exam (pupils, eye movements, nystagmus, fundoscopic exam, etc.) can be learned from Chapters 5 and 6 of this text. However, palsies of CNs III and VI are of particular interests to the neurosurgeon. A CN III palsy can have two components: (1) dysfunction of the outer parasympathetic fibers that supply the ciliary muscles and the pupillary sphincter, which would manifest as a dilated pupil ("fixed and dilated"); and (2) dysfunction of the levator palpebrae muscle of the eyelid and four of the extraocular muscles (superior, middle, inferior recti, and inferior oblique), which would manifest as ptosis and an eye that is "down and out," in which the eye cannot be adducted and the lateral rectus and superior oblique are spared (CNs IV and VI).[11] The parasympathetic fibers that control pupillary constriction are located on the outside of the nerve. A fixed and dilated pupil is concerning to a neurosurgeon because it can point to a compressive lesion on the nerve itself, such as from a posterior communicating aneurysm or impending uncal herniation. The somatic fibers that control the motor components of the third nerve are located on the inner portions of the nerve and are more sensitive to ischemic changes of the nerve, such as from hypertension or diabetes. Patients who have a "pupil-sparing" third nerve palsy are less worrisome to the neurosurgery clinician because this suggests a more systemic problem rather than a lesion of the brain that is causing mass effect on the nerve.[8]

A CN VI palsy is seen as an eye that is laterally located (either partially or completely) and cannot be adducted. Although a CN VI palsy can have many etiologies, increased intracranial pressure (ICP) is the most dreaded cause. Due to the long and aberrant course of the nerve in the subarachnoid space, CN VI is very sensitive to increases in ICP.[12] Again, any dysfunction of either of these CNs warrants a head CT of the patient.

Strength exam

General strength exam

Table 12.4 shows the general neurosurgical strength exam. The strength exam via telecommunication will require an examiner to be with the patient. Each of the four extremities can be given a strength grade and can be specified as the "proximal" or "distal" portion extremity for concise

Table 12.4 General neurosurgical strength exam.

Extremity ability	Strength grade
No movement	0/5
Muscle twitch observed	1/5
Able to move extremity, but not against gravity	2/5
Able to move extremity against gravity, but not against resistance	3/5
Able to move extremity against minor resistance	4−/5
Able to move extremity against moderate resistance	4/5
Able to move extremity against severe resistance, but not full strength	4+/5
Full strength against resistance	5/5

communication. For example: "The patient's left upper extremity was 5/5 proximally, but only 3/5 distally." When more detail is desired, each muscle group of any extremity can be given a strength grade.

Pronator drift

Pronator drift, commonly referred to as just "drift," is an examination maneuver that is commonly assessed in any focused general neurosurgical exam. To perform a drift exam, ask the patient to close his/her eyes and to raise both arms against gravity at shoulder level, palms facing the ceiling for at least 10 s. A positive drift would be manifested as one extremity that slowly drifts downward, together with supination of the extremity, after a few seconds. A positive pronator drift can indicate a contralateral upper motor neuron dysfunction in the contralateral hemisphere.

Examination of the spine

Chapter 13 will discuss the many details of the neurosurgical examination of the spine.

The Babinski reflex

The Babinski reflex is a primitive reflex that is usually gone by 1 year of age. To elicit this reflex from a remote setting, another examiner would need to be with the patient. That examiner strokes the sole of the patient's foot with a blunt instrument beginning at the heel of the foot, then moving toward the toes in a single, continuous curve. A normal, adult response manifests as a flexor plantar response (the toes pointing downwards); an abnormal adult response manifests as an extensor plantar response (the toes point upwards and flailing outward). Typically, for ease of communication, neurosurgery clinicians communicate a normal reflex as the patient having a "down-going response" to the Babinski maneuver, and an abnormal reflex as the patient having an "up-going response" to the Babinski maneuver. The Babinski reflex tests the integrity of the corticospinal tract (CST). The CST is a descending fiber tract that originates from the cerebral cortex through the brainstem and spinal cord. Fibers from the CST synapse with the alpha motor neuron in the spinal cord and help direct motor function. The CST is considered the upper motor neuron (UMN) and the alpha motor neuron is considered the lower motor neuron (LMN). Sixty percent of the CST fibers originate from the primary motor cortex, premotor areas, and supplementary motor areas. The remainder originates from primary sensory areas, the parietal cortex, and the operculum. An up-going Babinski reflex designates damage to the corticospinal tract (upper motor neuron damage). Damage anywhere along the CST can result in the presence of a Babinski sign.[13]

Sensory exam

A thorough sensory exam consists of assessment of light tough, pain and temperature, vibration, and proprioception. Each of these components requires an examiner to be with the patient if interviewing a patient via telecommunication. Chapter 13 will discuss the intricacies of the sensory exam for the extremities. The Romberg test is assessed by having the patient stand with the feet together and with his or her eyes closed. A "positive" Romberg sign is observed when the patient loses balance (someone should be with the patient to provide support in case this happens). This test helps to diagnose sensory ataxia, a gait disturbance caused by abnormal proprioception about the location of the joints; the test assesses the presence or absence of postural control without visual input suggestive of proprioceptive deficit in the lower limbs.[14,15]

Coordination

Dysfunction in coordination can have many etiologies in the brain; however, pathology from the cerebellum is the first thing that comes to mind for the practicing neurosurgeon.

Dysdiadochokinesia

Dysdiadochokinesia refers to the inability to perform rapid, alternating movements. The remote clinician should ask the patient to pat his or her hands on the thighs, alternating from the palm to the back of the hand (pronation and supination) as fast and as coordinated as possible. Dysdiadochokinesia is a form of cerebellar ataxia can result from vascular (e.g., stroke), toxic (e.g., alcoholism), or neoplastic (e.g., mass effect caused by a tumor), among many others.[16]

Dysmetria

Dysmetria refers to the inability to perform coordinated tasks. If another examiner is with the patient, the patient should be asked to perform the finger-to-nose test. The "finger-to-nose test" is performed by asking the patient to alternate from touching his or her nose to touching the index finger of the examiner as the examiner moves his or her own finger to and from various positions. If another examiner is not with the patient, the remote clinician can ask the patient to perform the "heel-to-shin" test. This test is performed by asking the patient to stroke the shin up and down, back and forth with the contralateral heel. Any interruption or difficulty with this task can be a sign of cerebellar dysmetria.

Conclusions

This chapter introduced the general neurosurgery exam for clinicians who are interested in implementing it in their telemedicine practice. The future of medicine is dependent on adapting to the current times. Interviewing and examining patients from a remote setting is, for better or worse, going to become more and more popular. It is pertinent that the field of medicine formulates new guidelines and published methods of the best practices of examining patients through telemedicine.

References

1. Knecht S, Dräger B, Deppe M, et al. Handedness and hemispheric language dominance in healthy humans. *Brain*. 2000;123(Pt 12):2512–2518.
2. McLernon S. The Glasgow Coma Scale 40 years on: a review of its practical use. *Br J Neurosci Nurs*. 2014;10(4):179–184. https://doi.org/10.12968/bjnn.2014.10.4.179.
3. Bilgin S, Guclu-Gunduz A, Oruckaptan H, Kose N, Celik B. Gait and Glasgow coma scale scores can predict functional recovery in patients with traumatic brain injury. *Neural Regen Res*. 2012;7(25):1978–1984. https://doi.org/10.3969/j.issn.1673-5374.2012.25.009.

4. Demetriades D, Kuncir E, Velmahos GC, Rhee P, Alo K, Chan LS. Outcome and prognostic factors in head injuries with an admission Glasgow coma scale score of 3. *Arch Surg.* 2004;139(10):1066–1068. https://doi.org/10.1001/archsurg.139.10.1066.

5. Lee JJ, Segar DJ, Asaad WF. Comprehensive assessment of isolated traumatic subarachnoid hemorrhage. *J Neurotrauma.* 2014;31(7):595–609. https://doi.org/10.1089/neu.2013.3152.

6. Jain S, Iverson LM. Glasgow coma scale. In: *StatPearls [Internet].* Treasure Island, FL: StatPearls Publishing; 2020.

7. Duncan R, Thakore S. Decreased Glasgow coma scale score does not mandate endotracheal intubation in the emergency department. *J Emerg Med.* 2009;37(4):451–455. https://doi.org/10.1016/j.jemermed.2008.11.026.

8. Agarwal P, Zhang DY, Grady MS. Neurological examination. In: *Neurosurgery Fundamentals.* Thieme Medical Publishers; 2018:23–39.

9. Acharya AB, Wroten M. Broca aphasia. In: *StatPearls [Internet].* Treasure Island, FL: StatPearls Publishing; 2020.

10. Acharya AB, Wroten M. Wernicke aphasia. In: *StatPearls [Internet].* StatPearls Publishing; 2020.

11. Modi P, Cranial AT. Nerve III palsy. In: *StatPearls [Internet]*; 2020.

12. Graham C, Mohseni M. Abducens Nerve (CN VI) palsy. In: *StatPearls [Internet]*; 2020.

13. Acharya AB, Jamil RT, Dewey JJ. Babinski reflex. In: *StatPearls [Internet].* Treasure Island, FL: StatPearls Publishing; 2020.

14. Lanska DJ, Goetz CG. Romberg's sign: development, adoption, and adaptation in the 19th century. *Neurology.* 2000;55(8):1201–1206. https://doi.org/10.1212/WNL.55.8.1201.

15. Galán-Mercant A, Cuesta-Vargas AI. Mobile Romberg test assessment (mRomberg). *BMC Res Notes.* 2014;7(1):1–8. https://doi.org/10.1186/1756-0500-7-640.

16. Rocha Cabrero F, De Jesus O. Dysdiadochokinesia. In: *StatPearls [Internet].* Treasure Island, FL: StatPearls Publishing; 2020.

Neurosurgical spine care during COVID-19 pandemic: The Department of Neurological Surgery Houston Methodist experience

Fernando E. Silva, MD[a], Gavin W. Britz, MD, MPH, MBA, FAANS[b], Paul Holman, MD[a,b]

[a]Director of Neurosurgical Spine Center and Director of Neurosurgical Spine Fellowship Program, Neurological Surgery, Houston Methodist Hospital, Houston, TX, United States
[b]Department of Neurosurgery, Houston Methodist Hospital, Houston, TX, United States

Introduction

Telemedicine has traditionally been utilized for remote consultations in areas of medicine such as trauma, neurology, and psychiatry.[1] However, with the 2020 COVID-19 pandemic, multiple disciplines of medicine quickly learned the utility of this modality of providing health care to our patients. This became necessary in order to deliver health care during this pandemic while reducing staff exposure to ill persons, reducing the burden of cases, as well as preserving personal protective equipment. Although this presented some challenges, namely changing some of our traditional ways of assessing patients, we saw this as a great opportunity not only to learn, but also to continue to provide neurosurgical spine care to our existing patients as well as to offer health care to new patients.

Our approach

The approach began with communicating to our established patients that continuity of care was available through telemedicine. The referring physicians were made aware of our capacity to offer telemedicine evaluation to new patients. Prior to the pandemic, a physician had to be licensed in the state where the patient was located; however, waivers were put in place to allow physicians to serve some patients out of state. We did not face this situation, as most of our patients remained in the state of Texas.[2]

The process also was easier to implement immediately as non-Health Insurance Portability and Accountability Act (HIPPA)-compliant modes of communication, such as FaceTime, became permissible. Hence, the option was given to the patient to communicate via video teleconferencing, including FaceTime, telephone only, or electronic communication such as email. Almost unanimously, our patient population elected for video teleconferencing, and we used HIPPA-compliant teleconferencing means of communication, using electronic privacy information center (EPIC) electronic medical record (Verona, Wisconsin). Only on the rare occasion of being unable to connect, after multiple attempts, did we conduct the evaluation via telephone. We did not find it necessary ever to employ electronic communication by way of email or medical record messaging, except for sending out and receiving new patient packet information. Once the patient was scheduled for a visit, the workflow essentially followed the same pattern as for our face-to-face inpatient visits.

The visit

Most of our follow-ups, including postoperative, scheduled, and new patients, agreed to telemedicine follow-up/consultation. The typical patient packet information was emailed to new patients. The latter was then reviewed within 30 min prior to their appointment by our medical assistant, especially the patient's mode of identification, chief complaint, onset, location, duration, and previous treatment of symptoms, medication allergies, and current medications. Once this was completed, the medical assistant instructed the patient to log onto the mode of communication chosen—EPIC EMR in our case—no less than 15 min prior to their scheduled appointment.

Evaluation/examination

For the appointment, patients were instructed to be in a quiet room and wearing comfortable clothing. At this point the visit was no different than in-person visits, beginning with a detailed history taking, addressing each pertinent symptom. Our examination was conducted in as detailed a manner as the mode of communication permitted (see Table 13.1). It was helpful during the examination to ask the patient to step away from the device so as to be able to see the entire body or ask somebody, such as a family member, to hold the device during the examination. In this fashion we were typically able to complete a mental status evaluation, cranial nerves

Table 13.1 Basic evaluation/examination.

	Face-to-face visit	Telemedicine
General appearance	Whether patient is well kept or not. Note any degree of distress.	Same
HEENT (head, eyes, ears, nose, and throat)	Look for any gross head trauma. Cervical range of movement. Pupillary function and funduscopic examination.	Look for any gross head trauma. Cervical range of movement.
Range of movement	Lumbar spine flexion extension, rotation, and lateral flexion	Same
Gait	Check whether gait unstable, antalgic or not	Same
Neurological	Orientation to self, place, and time	Same
Cranial nerves	II–XII: the usual manner	II (ask patient to read newspaper at arm's-length) VII (ask if patient is wearing hearing aids) IX (ask if patient has any difficulty with swallowing and note their phonation) Other CNs: the usual manner.
Motor function	Perform Barre. Motor strength graded 0–5 upper and lower extremity major muscle groups.	Perform Barre. Observe patient move all extremities against gravity and lift different weight objects. Ask patient to walk on heels and toes.
Cerebellar function	Note any nystagmus. Check finger-nose-finger testing and rapid alternating movements as well as heel-to-shin.	Same
Wound	Inspect for discharge, induration, and erythema	Same

assessment, limited motor exam, range of motion, cerebellar examination, gait, overall spinal balance, and wound assessment, on postoperative patients (Table 13.1).

Reviewing the patient's radiographic imaging with them was conducted by holding Kemmerer today patient is 30, such as CT scans, MRIs or reports of such as nerve conduction studies. In terms of acquiring the patient study, this was done either by having the patient delivered a compact disc to the clinic, or if the study was performed in our institution, simply looking it up in their electronic medical record. The CD data were then uploaded into our LifeImage (Newton, Massachusetts) and transferred to a picture archiving computer system (PACS); in this way we were able to share with the patient the salient study findings. If the study was already in our hospital system, it was simply opened in PACS and reviewed. Other studies such as dual energy x-ray absorptiometry (DEXA) scans and electromyography (EMGs)/nerve conduction velocity (NCVs) were reviewed and discussed during the visit. This approach was extremely useful in conveying findings to the patients and allowing them to ask question about the findings.

Diagnosis

During neurospine care telemedicine evaluation, certain diagnoses can be deciphered through history alone. For instance, one can reasonably accurately arrive at a diagnosis of cervical and lumbar radiculopathies, cervical myelopathy, and neurogenic claudication, based on the history and pain diagrams.[3,4] Additionally, physical findings such as antalgic gait and difficulty with heel/toe ambulation can help diagnose certain cases of lumbar disc herniation and myelopathy, respectively. In spinal deformity cases, evaluating for shoulder imbalance, trunk shift, lumbar crease, pelvic level, and gross assessment of the sagittal and coronal imbalance are easily evaluated via telemedicine. One simply asks the patient to stand with knees completely extended on a level floor, undressed to their underwear. At this point the camera is brought in front of the patient focusing on the shoulders, and it is noted if one shoulder is higher than the other. The camera is then brought to the back and the trunk asymmetry is assessed by noting if it is shifted to one side or the other relative to the head. Lumbar creases/skin folds are then noted to evaluate for any lumbar and lumbo-pelvic deformities, respectively. The Adam's forward bending test can then be performed by asking the patient to bend at the hips, and the axis of the camera is directed parallel to the thoracic cage first, then at the thoracolumbar/lumbar spine, noting any thoracic and thoracolumbar/lumbar rotation, respectively. This spinal

Table 13.2 Basic diagnosis.

	Face-to-face visit	Telemedicine
Radiculopathy/ myelopathy	Ask patient to show limb pain pattern and confirm by reviewing pain pattern diagram with them. Check Lermitt's and Spurling's.	Same
Lower back pain	Check if pain is elicited on flexion, extension, palpate lumbar facet, sacroiliac (SI), and hip joints. Check for pain on internal/external hip rotation.	Ask patient to: Flex and extend at the lumbar region while standing; internal/external rotate the hip while sitting.
Deformity	Observe shoulder level, trunk position, lumbar crease, pelvic level. Look for sagittal and coronal imbalance with the hips and knees fully extended.	Same

deformity assessment can help determine—along with the radiographic data, including scoliosis views—whether the patient needs treatment or not; if the latter, the patient may be advised regarding other treatment modalities (Table 13.2).

In this fashion, we were able to document a clinic note that was as accurate and complete as possible. Additionally, we found it useful to conclude such notes with this sentence:

Given the nature of our consultation via telemedicine today, a full exam is not permissible and I would like to see the patient in approximately [X] days/weeks for formal follow-up and examination.

Treatment

Any prescription for schedule II–V controlled substances was completed in the usual fashion, as well as for any prescriptions pertinent to their diagnosis.[5] When elective spine surgery was considered, this was discussed and spine models were brought to the camera to facilitate further discussion/explanation of the operation. At the end of the visit, the patients were scheduled for in-person follow-up as soon as feasible, particularly to conduct complete physical assessment, and to discuss further any surgical recommendations, as well as preoperative planning, pre- and postoperative care, and follow-up. Although there is no clear literature that we are aware of, preoperative screening, postoperative wound care, or general evaluation can be conducted by the supervised nurse practitioner and/or physician assistant, no different than in the usual face-to-face visit, provided adequate training has been given. We feel the latter fosters efficacy in term of the surgeon's schedule and keeps the practice productive, perhaps increasing the referral base, as some surgeons might not participate in a telemedicine-type practice.

Limits of telemedicine

Although we were able to continue to deliver care for patients with spinal conditions for stable, nonemergent conditions, one of the limitations of this mode of health care delivery is the inability to do so for those in need of urgent and emergent care. In such situations, in-person visits were continued through our emergency department services. Older patients requiring spine care might not be technically savvy enough to conduct a telemedicine visit, and without the help of family members, the visit might not be possible. Additionally, in spite of patients being able to use their devices such as tablets, phones, and computers, connectivity issues can limit the appropriateness of the visit. Finally, some patients might not be comfortable with this mode of health care delivery, and their cultural bias may play a role in the appropriateness of telemedicine health care delivery for spine care in these rare situations.

Conclusion

In our practice, telemedicine during the COVID-19 pandemic proved to be an excellent way to continue caring for our established patients and to evaluate new patients, particularly those with nonemergent spine issues. Most of our follow-up and scheduled patients were able to keep their initial appointments. This helped us to avoid any significant backlog in terms of health care delivery. Although we do not see telemedicine as a global approach to neurosurgical spine care, it has, particularly in situations such as the COVID-19 pandemic, proven to be a useful tool for different medical disciplines; as such, telemedicine will continue to be helpful and used in our practice, as it can also improve patient health outcomes.[6] However, to the latter end, it is imperative that insurance carriers, as well as Medicare and Medicaid, continue to allow reimbursement for telemedicine visits.[7] Life presents us with many changes and challenges, and caring for patients during the COVID-19 pandemic has been no different. We have not only learned immensely, but feel that we have delivered compassionate and responsible health care to our spine patients, even in the face of these challenges.

References

1. Latifi R, Dogiani A, Dasho E, et al. Telemedicine former trauma in Albania: initial results from case series of 146 patients. *World Neurosurg.* 2018;112:e747–e753.
2. Wright JH, Caudill R. Remote treatment delivery in response to COVID-19 pandemic. *Psychother Psychosom.* 2020;89(3):130–132.
3. Matz PG, Anderson PA, Kaiser MG, et al. Introduction and methodology: guidelines for the surgical management of cervical degenerative disease. *J Neurosurg Spine.* 2009;11:101–103.
4. Jason, C. Eck et al. Guideline update for the performance of fusion procedures for degenerative disc disease of the lumbar spine. *J Neurosurg.* 2014;21:1–139.
5. Silva FE, Lenke LG. Adult degenerative scoliosis: evaluation and management. *Neurosurg Focus.* 2010;28(3):E1.
6. O'Connor M, Asdornwised U, Dempsey ML, et al. Using telehealth to reduce all-because 30-day hospital readmissions and known heart failure patient is receiving skilled home health services. *Plan Clin Inform.* 2016;7(2):238–247.
7. Medicare and Medicaid Programs. *Policy and regulatory revisions in response to COVID-19 public health emergency;* 2020.

CHAPTER 14

System coordination and implementation

John J. Volpi, MD
Director of Stroke Division, Houston Methodist Neurological Institute, Houston Methodist Hospital, Houston, TX, United States

In this chapter, we explore the concept of a system of care for telemedicine through three cases that illustrate the challenges of expansion. Whether virtual or traditional, a system of care is necessary to provide comprehensive services throughout a health care setting. But what is a system of care? A system of care is the whole environment of individuals and resources that surround a patient and the processes that coordinate those individuals and resources. A useful example is that of a patient with a seizure. We can see how a system of care begins when the patient collapses at home and 911 is called. The system of care for this patient would include the county 911 dispatcher who alerts EMS (emergency medical services) that a seizure patient needs help, and the EMS personnel who arrive and transport the patient to a local emergency department (ED) capable of handling an unstable, possibly intubated patient. From there, the system of care includes the ED physician, who may be concerned enough about status epilepticus that he or she contacts an affiliated tertiary facility with 24/7 neurophysiology to take the patient in transfer. Once stable, the tertiary facility may further expand the system by involving a subspecialty epileptologist for clinic follow-up and possibly even a neurosurgeon who specializes in epilepsy surgery. In this example, the patient simply called 911 and depended on the health care system to be responsive and efficient in coordinating the best care. From the system standpoint, protocols and properly trained personnel had to be developed, updated, and coordinated to ensure the patient received the care.

While neurological patients may enter a health care system through a hospital admission, they are often seen by family doctors and referred to specialty care. This too is a system of care, but one that often has fewer protocols and less coordination. In many parts of the US and the world, neurology appointments can be difficult to schedule due to limited availability.

Even some hospitals may not have full-time neurology coverage, and even fewer have routine access to subspecialists, such as an epileptologist, as in the example above.

A major strength of telemedicine is its utility across many different care settings to bridge gaps that are apparent in more traditional models. New clinic visits, emergency department encounters, follow-up visits, and subspecialty opinion visits allow expertise to reach patients through telemedicine despite geographic and resource barriers. Some counties are even implementing telemedicine services in ambulances. Realizing this strength of telemedicine, many institutions are seeking ways to cooperate among members of their own organization and leverage expertise where it is needed and when it is needed. The specific example of telestroke coverage to deliver vascular neurology care to the ED is only the beginning of a spectrum of possibilities for connecting the right patient to the right doctor. For physicians, the appeal of such arrangements is that they allow the practice both to grow and to become more focused.

Before exploring the case studies, it is worthwhile first considering the conceptual arrangement for a system. Often it is suggested that systems have spokes and one or more hubs. While this is familiar and a simple, useful arrangement for some systems, it often does not capture the real-world needs of most institutions. Furthermore, in neurology the spokes may evoke the image of a general neurologist, and while a true "general neurologist" may occasionally exist, even a generalist typically has a practice focus or prior training that makes him or her better suited for a subset of patients that is distinct from another colleague who also practices general neurology.

More problematic, a spoke and hub arrangement evokes a sense of superior-inferior, which can undercut system progress and collegiality. Most systems of care have a wide variety of clinics, freestanding facilities, and hospitals that do not neatly fit into a spoke or a hub. They may not even fit into the same umbrella institution. A clinic on the east side of town may have an autonomic testing lab, while a facility on the west side of town may perform muscle biopsies, and yet another may share space with a private neuro-ophthalmologist. Are these spokes or hubs? How then should we consider such a system? The better analogy is a wide array of various-sized gears. Gears depend on each other to move and when one moves the others react; unfortunately, if one breaks, the whole system becomes vulnerable. Some gears may be small, others large, but the cooperative nature of this arrangement better illustrates the true variety of facilities and physician practices that combine to form a system.

Core values should guide decisions

On the surface, systems of care may share a logo or a balance sheet, but what really unites a system is its shared values.[1] If a system values excellence in neurosciences, it will be more likely to invest in teleneurology services, but regardless of any system's priority for neuroscience excellence, there are two core values that must be in place for a system:

(1) a commitment to cooperative growth; and

(2) recognition of the fiduciary role to patients.

A commitment to cooperative growth is a fundamental feature of a successful system of care. Actions that undercut trust, ignore stakeholders, or direct services for purely financial gain will ultimately lead to inefficient systems.[2]

The fiduciary role of the health care professional is to put the patient's needs ahead of their own. Such clear principles are easy to discern when one considers a single patient, but may become less clear when a collective, future group of patients are considered. Nonetheless, the obligation to put the patient first does not change and must also remain a core feature of the system of care.

In the next three sections, we will examine actual challenges or outright conflicts that arose in developing a system of care for telemedicine in a mixed urban, suburban, and rural environment. In each case, the scenario may seem familiar or may differ from those encountered in your own environment, but they were chosen to highlight pitfalls that can be avoided with strategic, thoughtful planning. As a reader, consider taking a moment after each case to jot down the source of the problem and potential solutions—the more the better. In considering the various solutions, be mindful of the fiduciary role of the system as well as the need for cooperative growth. Are these core principles served? How is the conflict a reflection of misguided actions? After each case, a discussion will follow that explores how things went wrong and then how solutions came to be. No one answer is correct and the most important takeaway is the process of planning itself.

Case 1: Dr. Garcia needs help at the hospital

Dr. Garcia is a general neurologist who practices in a rural clinic that is part of the St. Elizabeth System of Hospitals (StESH). Adjacent to the clinic is a 75-bed hospital that is a primary stroke center and serves a population of about 25,000 people. The clinic and hospital where Dr. Garcia works was previously part of Unity Healthcare and was purchased 2 years ago by StESH, which now owns eight regional hospitals and employees a group of 700 physicians. The StESH Main Campus has 15 neurologists and a new teleneurology service that is currently operating at two of the eight hospitals in the StESH system but not at Dr. Garcia's hospital. Dr. Garcia joined the employed practice with an agreement to do five night/weekend calls per month. The remainder of the hospital calls would be covered by a private group of physicians who are paid a per diem rate and were part of the Unity Hospital but opted not to join StESH. The typical neurology census at the hospital is about 5–10 patients, with two or three new consults per day.

Dr. Garcia has an interest in expanding her hospital consults. She feels that she could see all of the hospital patients every weekday and at least one weekend per month. Although she did not do a fellowship in vascular neurology, she enjoys caring for stroke patients and has kept up with the latest advancements in thrombectomy and imaging for stroke patients.

In addition to building her practice, she has some concerns that the private group rotates providers too frequently and the lack of continuity of care for patients has caused some lapses in quality. The hospital CEO supports her decision and would also like to hire more StESH neurologists, but his neuroscience budget is limited due to the per diem he is paying the private group.

Dr. Garcia asks the CEO to come up with a plan to cover after hours and weekend call with teleneurology and she will provide in person rounds on the patients. The CEO discusses teleneurology with Dr. Randolph, a provider at StESH Main Campus who coordinates teleneurology. Dr. Randolph and the CEO negotiate a plan that costs the CEO 50% of his prior per diem budget and allows him to invest in another neurologist for the practice in time. The CEO informs Dr. Garcia that she can see the patients during the day and Dr. Randolph's team will cover acute issues after hours and weekend.

Questions to consider for Case 1

1. Who are the stakeholders in the plan to add teleneurology to the call schedule?
2. What pitfalls might exist with the plan?
3. Are the goals of patient care and growth presently aligned, and does the current plan improve or worsen the alignment of these goals?

Discussion

One of the most common mistakes made in putting together a system of care is inadvertently forgetting important stakeholders.[3] In this case, an accommodating CEO, an ambitious local neurologist, and a well-organized telemedicine team made a plan without the input of many other members of the system of care. A critical first step in planning a system of care for telemedicine is identifying stakeholders. The list in this case might include the emergency department physicians and nurses, the county EMS chief, hospitalist physicians, the nursing director for the stroke center, the other system hospitals that are still not served by the teleneurology service, and the private practice that has long served the hospital before it was part of StESH and continues to provide call coverage 25 out of 30 days.

An alienated stakeholder can derail a well-intentioned plan. In this case, the CEO informed the private group that he would be ending the per diem pay but welcomed their ongoing presence at the hospital. Feeling left out of the decision-making process, they informed the CEO that they would not see patients at the hospital any longer and would no longer provide coverage as part of a call pool, leaving the hospital with Dr. Garcia as the lone neurologist on staff.

The emergency department physicians initially liked the idea of a teleneurology service, but became concerned when the hospitalist physicians did not want to admit unstable neurological patients without a plan from a staff neurologist whom they could easily contact. The floor nurses were unsure who to call with questions overnight and did not have any setups for video visits like the ED had. The hospitalists requested significantly more patients with neurological complaints transfer to Main Campus. Patients and their families who were accustomed to care at the local hospital found themselves transferred 30 miles and having to drive an hour to Main Campus to see their family. Recognizing this trend, EMS started diverting more stroke and seizure calls to other hospitals and bypassing the StESH campus. With a shrinking neuroscience patient population, the CEO no longer had the budget available to hire a second employed neurologist. Dr. Garcia also felt left out of the call pool for teleneurology and had expected Dr. Randolph to include her in the rotation of telemedicine providers.

Solutions and realignment

In reality, the plan did not unravel as spectacularly as described, mostly because the hospital CEO was astute enough to recognize the stakeholders during a soft introduction and series of meetings where many of these issues came to light.

Dr. Randolph met with Dr. Garcia and explained that the budget for the current year of teleneurology service had already been allocated, but that he welcomed her interest and offered to have her shadow a few nights of call to see if it was something she would like to join in the future.

The ED medical director took the lead in working with his providers and the hospitalists to ensure that unstable patients would be given extra scrutiny before transferring to a floor bed and that they would utilize more intermediate units and intensive care unit (ICU) beds when there was any lingering concern about a patient's stability. Dr. Randolph also met with the ICU team and hospitalists and reassured them that the teleneurology physician would be available throughout the initial hospital course to manage any issues even outside the ED until the in-person neurologist saw the patient. The teleneurologists provided the nursing staff with a single hotline to reach the on-call teleneurologist and a set of iPads for video encounters. Dr. Randolph and the ED medical director also met with the local EMS chief and explained that in similar rollouts, the utilization of tPA (tissue plasminogen activator) increased, and shared literature that showed how a successful prehospital notification of the teleneurology team would further shrink door-to-needle times. This partnership was well received by the EMS, which had been interested in enhancing prehospital stroke scores.

As for the private group, the CEO recognized that they would be taking a financial loss and decided a phased approach would be better than a cold break. He offered the private team a 50% reduction in per diem rates, recognizing that their services would still be needed but their afterhours responsibilities were significantly less. They agreed to this plan for 1 year. The total amount the hospital was paying for neurology call was the same for 1 year but would be split between teleneurology and in-person call pay. While there were ultimately no call pay savings in the first year, the volume of patients grew, and the CEO was able to justify a new hire.

Takeaways

When treating patients, physicians are well attuned to the downstream effects of their therapies. An antiplatelet medication reduces stroke risk but may cause a gastrointestinal bleed. An antiseizure medicine may stop seizures but cause excessive sleepiness and imbalance. While the physician is accustomed to the chess game of thinking two steps ahead physiologically, the same planning and careful consideration must apply to make changes within a system. In almost every telemedicine system of care, change will result in collateral effects. Change itself can be a source of resistance for no other reason than it is different from how things have always been done.[4]

When facing these challenges, it can be disheartening to hear a barrage of complaints about a well-intentioned plan. The remedy for such criticism is to listen early and often and to plan over time based on this feedback.[5] To engage stakeholders, start with any point of stress in the system and hold listening sessions. In this case, Dr. Garcia meeting with the ED medical director would be a sensible early contact. For these meetings, it is best not to have a specific plan or even agenda. By listening and addressing concerns, one can turn stakeholders into champions. These champions may be formal leaders, but in any department there are also informal leaders who may not have a specific leadership title in the organization, but who play an outsized role in the organization's morale. These may be long-tenured staff, or personal friends of the leaders, or just very vocal individuals whose disagreement can sink a plan. These individuals are key allies to bring into the fold early to avoid demoralizing backchannel criticism.

When facing difficult changes, such as the CEO informing the private team of a pay cut, make a point of holding in-person meetings that emphasize the values of the organization and frankly address how the environment is changing. While email may be efficient, it is the worst possible vehicle for introducing difficult changes. The CEO should find out how important the per diem call pay is for the private practice, and point out that as fewer and fewer neurologists want to take overnight acute calls, he must make forward-looking and patient-centered plans that are appropriate for the future.

Many courses and lectures exist on change management, and the details are outside the scope of this chapter but included as references at the end.[4] Experienced health care executives are well-versed in change management and can be valuable colleagues in navigating a plan through resistance.

Finally, it is important to remember the core values of putting the patient first and cooperative growth. While these values may seem simple, they increase dramatically in complexity as more and more stakeholders face a change to the status quo.

Case 2: The call volume is increasing

Dr. Randolph has started a successful teleneurology program at StESH. For the first 6 months, he covered all the calls himself from just one campus. He now has three of the eight campuses participating and has received enough funding to recruit a full-time faculty member and cover half of their salary with telemedicine revenue. He has also been able to fund call pay for two more of his colleagues to participate. The panel of teleneurologists taking acute calls now includes four faculty members with experience in acute neurological care.

The program has been very well received by the ED providers, who appreciate the rapid response and video evaluations. As a result, the program has had an increase in calls over the last 24 months, as shown in Fig. 14.1.

In order to manage the increasing call volume, Dr. Randolph has made a number of presentations to the ED physicians and nurses on best practices. He has heard complaints from his three other providers that the "ER calls for everything" and "If the patient is stable, they should hold the consult for the day team." On the other side, he has had two complaints in the last month that one of his providers, Dr. Davis, was rude to an ED secretary and nurse. For his part, Dr. Davis has written a few emails to the ED directors, the most recent with the subject line: "PLEASE REVIEW PROPER USE OF ACUTE ACTIVATIONS!"

Dr. Randolph understands the stress of overnight calls and, after the latest email, took Dr. Davis out of the call pool for 2 weeks to give him a rest, but consequently, Dr. Randolph and the rest of the pool shared an increased burden of calls in addition to their full-time faculty responsibilities.

Dr. Randolph feels strongly that teleneurology is the right answer for providing additional services and has encouraged his pool of providers by

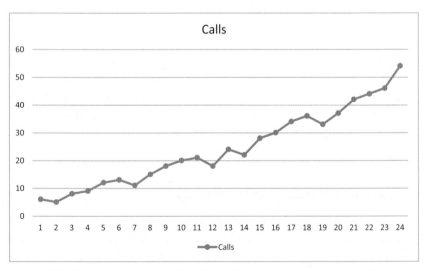

Fig. 14.1 Growth in number of after-hour calls to the teleneurology service line.

providing a night call rate that is generous and welcome as they had not received any compensation for Main Campus calls in the past.

Questions to consider for Case 2

1. Is the current model scalable for the growth the acute teleneurology service line is experiencing?
2. What factors are contributing to the friction between the ED providers and the teleneurology providers?
3. What solutions might be best for easing the concerns of the teleneurology call pool?

Discussion

Dr. Randolph was concerned that his team was putting forth more effort now that the call volume was increasing and the pay for the call was no longer aligned with their effort. He reviewed the budget and had expected a fourth center to start in the next quarter. Looking at the increase in funding, he found he could provide a 30% increase in the call pay to the pool. He presented the new rates to the team and overall the reception was enthusiastic. One member of the pool, Dr. Warren, commented that the raise was in line with what her colleagues at a private company "Neurologist on Duty" were being paid and they were often up all night. She felt it was a fair deal and reflected the market rates.

Dr. Davis had also just bought a new house and commented that "every dollar counts" now in his life, and he was feeling good about the pay raise. Dr. Randolph was glad to see Dr. Davis motivated to remain on the team and felt his earlier dissatisfaction should be allayed with the pay increase.

For the first month, the team had no disruptions, but by the second month, the situation deteriorated. Dr. Warren had become pregnant and was very nauseated and asked to reduce her calls to once per week. With the extra calls now turning into more sleepless nights, Dr. Davis became more insistent that Dr. Randolph take a hard line with the ED providers and start refusing calls unless the patient met clear criteria for acute evaluations. Despite his reluctance, Dr. Randolph agreed that if a patient did not meet criteria for acute evaluation, the teleneurologist could, at his or her discretion, defer a consult to the day team.

The night after this decision, Dr. Davis was on call and a unit secretary paged for a patient with 3 days of headache. Upon calling back at 2 a.m., Dr. Davis curtly informed the ED secretary that "There is no reason to wake me up at 2 a.m. for a headache patient. Tell the ED doctor that I am refusing this consult and Dr. Randolph will hear about this inappropriate activation in the morning and I'm filing a complaint with your medical staff for not following protocol!" The hospital's director of nursing reviewed the call and felt that Dr. Davis was out of line and was so angry with the doctor that she recommended he be temporarily removed from the staff until a full investigation could take place over 1–3 months.

Facing a further-reduced panel of providers, Dr. Randolph went to the hospital leadership and asked them to approach the "Neurologist on Duty" company for coverage. The leadership informed Dr. Randolph that even if a contract met their needs, it would take at least 90 days to formalize a deal and they would need to reduce his budget significantly.

Solutions and realignment

Although the situation did not become quite this dire in reality, the problem of burnout quickly became a concern. When Dr. Randolph started the program, he had many nights with zero calls and even a busy night was one or two calls. As the participating centers increased and ED providers changed their habits, there were no more easy calls and a typical night had four to six calls, often disrupting the providers' sleep to such a degree that it began having consequences for their mood and even health.

Physician burnout is topic of much discussion and the teleneurologist taking overnight call is particularly vulnerable.[6] The key error in judgment that Dr. Randolph made was expecting extra compensation to be a cure for dissatisfaction. Surveys across many industries including medicine show that compensation is not the most important factor in job satisfaction. Factors such as new challenges, a sense of purpose, appreciation for work, good relationship with colleagues, and work–life balance are typically the leading indicators of satisfaction and prevent burnout.[7]

In this case, the other fundamental error was a lapse in the fiduciary role to the patient. Although it may not have been clear to him at the time, Dr. Randolph and his panel were becoming increasingly exhausted and this exhaustion was turning into mental fatigue and higher risk of errors and poor decision-making. The patient's interest in having a competent, healthy, focused provider should come first and ahead of any programmatic goals for Dr. Randolph to grow the service or the providers to earn extra pay.

In the example of Dr. Davis's refusal, the facts of the case were never presented. Out of frustration, Dr. Davis assumed the patient had a benign headache but never actually asked important questions of the ED provider to ensure that the headache did not have serious features such as meningismus or explosive onset, or that the patient had any history of trauma. Dr. Davis was experienced and respected by his colleagues and this behavior was clearly a result of exhaustion.[8]

Before the situation reached this point, the administrator working with Dr. Randolph had a frank discussion with him. The administrator explained that no amount of pay would fix the problems the program was facing. Together they came up with a strategy to hire a nocturnist with the extra funds and keep the call pay the same for the time being. They found a neurologist who was well qualified and had a physical disability as a result of a recent, serious injury that prevented her from walking. The idea of restoring her purpose as a physician, being part of something new, and growing the program while she was undergoing her own physical rehabilitation was very appealing and the nocturnist was enthusiastic on call.

As a result of having a nocturnist, Dr. Randolph's team had coverage for 20 out of 30 nights per month, leaving the pool two or three each per month. Dr. Randolph worked with the clinic staff to make sure that on these two or three postcall days the clinic volume was reduced for the providers and shifted to the afternoon so they could get some sleep before work.

Takeaways

The enthusiasm and excitement of starting a teleneurology program can provide satisfaction and personal momentum for many months, but eventually growth will require scaling up. For leaders who were heavily invested in the start-up phase, this scale up phase can be particularly difficult as it often requires changing the ways things are done and giving up control. Well-meaning leaders will see control as particularly important and forget the importance of cooperative growth. Knowing the program inside and out and having invested personal, often uncompensated time will lead to a strong desire to stay the course even if it means an unrealistic and unsustainable burden on oneself and colleagues. The early momentum can turn into unhealthy inertia.[9]

During the growth phase of a teleneurology system, a useful exercise for a program is to consider a leadership strategy meeting or retreat. Multiple resources exist to review risks and remedies for burnout, and references are provided at the end of this chapter. Simply taking a breather from the day in and day out, and talking about the challenges, may be enough to recognize that growth means change and sharing control. Most physicians recognize the importance of work-life balance but may fail to recognize when it is slowly eroding.

Early hires in a program are likely to be through personal contacts and well-established credentials, but as a program grows, it will need to recruit through more sophisticated and sustainable means. There are many creative options available for covering nights including overseas partnerships or reaching out to providers on temporary leave for life reasons or disabilities. In addition, as teleneurology programs grow in nearby regions, opportunities for sharing calls across systems may arise. These calls may be busier but less frequent, a trade-off that most teleneurologists who are maintaining a regular daytime practice will appreciate. In some cases, a contractual relationship to a private pool of providers may also be a good option.

Ultimately, burnout remains one of the major threats to the success of any system of care and especially a teleneurology practice relying on overnight work. Recognizing the deleterious effect it has on patient care, physician health, and long-term program goals is as crucial as refocusing a program as it grows on a strategy that can sustain lasting value.

Case 3: System-wide adoption

After a successful rollout at four of the eight StESH hospitals, Dr. Randolph has asked the council of CEOs to adopt a plan that would provide telemedicine across the entire eight hospital system over the next year. Dr. Randolph has made personal visits to each hospital, met with the CEOs, ED medical directors, and stroke directors, and feels that telemedicine is an important part of system-based standardization of care.

He reviews the budget with his administrator and presents a hiring plan to staff the teleneurology division over the ramp-up phase of the next 12 months.

The remaining four hospitals are as follows:

StESH North has 300 beds and services a diverse patient population in middle-income suburbs. The hospital has a stroke medical director, Dr. Warren, who shares traditional acute call with a mix of private and employed physicians. Dr. Warren has also been serving on the pool of teleneurology providers for more than 1 year and would like to see her facility transition from a primary stroke center to a comprehensive stroke center. The CEO of StESH North is very interested in becoming a comprehensive stroke center as well.

StESH Far West is a rural hospital with 60 beds serving three small communities of mostly low- to middle-income communities. It is about 10 miles from a larger regional hospital that is not part of the StESH and is a primary stroke center. StESH Far West is not yet a primary stroke center and employs two predominantly outpatient neurologists who contribute 10 days total call per month and do a round every weekday. These two neurologists have fellowship training in epilepsy and movement disorders and have made it clear to their hospital leadership that they do not feel comfortable managing acute stroke patients. The hospital CEO currently has no plans to add another neurologist, but she would like to achieve primary stroke center status in the next 1–2 years.

StESH Coastal City is a new, 200-bed facility serving a high-income suburb. This facility is almost adjacent to two competing hospital system facilities, one of which is already a comprehensive stroke center and the other is planning to be comprehensive in the next 6–12 months. The CEO of StESH Coastal City has made it clear that he cannot compete in his market unless he becomes comprehensive. He has hired a staff including an interventional neurosurgeon, an interventional neurologist, and a neurocritical neurologist, as well as two clinic-based neurologists. The interventionalists are pushing for more EMS volume.

StESH Village is an 85-bed hospital that has been in its middle- to upper-income community since the 1950s. It was also originally part of a different health care system, where it was financially struggling as a general hospital. It was then purchased by a group of orthopedic surgeons, who planned to turn it into a surgery center, but later StESH negotiated a 60% purchase; 40% remained with the orthopedic group. As part of the agreement, the CEO developed a plan to make it a center of excellence for orthopedics and OB/GYN. The hospital is very popular in the community and has a strong reputation for attracting prominent doctors, including two private practice neurologists who have been in practice for 30+ years at the Village Hospital. As a result, its ER volume is considerably higher than other facilities of similar size.

The facilities are summarized in Table 14.1.

Table 14.1 Summary of facilities.

StESH facility	North	Far west	Coastal city	Village
Beds	300	60	200	85
Stroke center?	Primary	No status	Opened as primary	No status
Other initiatives	Seeking comprehensive stroke status soon?	Would like to be primary	Seeking comprehensive status now	Ortho and OB/GYN centers of excellence
Staff neurologists	Six, mixed employed and private	Two employed, not interested in stroke call	All employed: two interventionalists, one neurocritical care, two clinic based	Two private practice with 30 + years at the hospital

Questions to consider for Case 3

1. What are some barriers for coordinating care across this system?
2. What factors should influence the budget requests from each facility to fund the teleneurology service?
3. Who are potential champions of a system-wide rollout?

Discussion

Dr. Randolph presents the CEO council with a two-tiered system for providing teleneurology service afterhours and on weekends. For hospitals that have fewer than 150 beds, the daily fee is half that of the hospitals with more than 150 beds. He explains that with the extra funding he will maintain a full-time nocturnist and hire a quality manager and an additional faculty member.

The Far West CEO is interested in the program but raises a concern that if her hospital wants to accept more stroke patients and become a primary stroke center, she will need coverage during the day as well as afterhours. If she could have such a plan, she would be interested, but she has no interest in afterhours only.

The North CEO finds the proposal acceptable but wants to know if Dr. Warren will be "double dipping" on the days she takes traditional call as well as teleneurology call at his facility. He thinks if she does get paid for both services simultaneously, his compliance department would reject the plan.

The Coastal City CEO also is interested in having the service since comprehensive stroke status will require vascular expertise every day and he currently only has it half the time. His concern is that he already pays for an on-call interventionalist as well as traditional in-person call, and he is unsure if he can pay for a third call pool.

The Village CEO thinks it is a "nice to have" but feels her hospital does not need such a service as it is exploring more of a niche market and has been profitable in this approach. She also thinks it may alienate her long-standing private practice neurologists who are well regarded by the staff and community, and who provide essentially all the coverage she needs.

Somewhat frustrated by the discussion at the meeting, Dr. Randolph shows statistics and economic data that support the value of a teleneurology program. Ultimately, the CEOs agree that it is a worthwhile goal, but may be better for next year's budget unless Dr. Randolph can rework the plan.

Solutions and realignment

As a system of care grows, an important question at times to ask is: what is the actual need that telemedicine serves that is not already served?[10] In this case, Dr. Randolph was growing a one-size-fits-all type of program. His program provided afterhours/weekend coverage, and while he had built in some flexibility on pricing, he had missed the bigger issue of flexibility in needs.

Often is it the need that comes first and then a program arises to fill it, but when growing a telemedicine system of care, it may be that once early needs are filled at some facilities, remaining parts of the system have much softer demand for the service.[11] If this is the case, it is important to turn the question back to the system and get guidance on what should be controlled from the top down and what should be locally controlled. Some of the most top-down systems are centrally controlled health care systems from counties or the Veterans Affairs (VA) health care system. In these cases, a central planning authority decides which facilities will be motherships and which will be feeders. Rolling out a telemedicine service to all facilities in this environment may be straightforward once the guidance is in place.

In private health care systems in the US, the market often drives the decisions.[12] In this case, Coastal City may not be filling a gap in their community, but instead trying to stay competitive with other providers in the region and the community's expectations. On the other hand, Far West and Village seem to be fulfilling profitable niches, but leaving their community with relatively less coverage.

Recognizing the disparity in needs and role of market forces, Dr. Randolph met with the CEO council a second time and listened to their needs.[13] He also explained that while he could adapt the current model to some degree, every patient across the system should have the expectation of the same, excellent quality of care no matter the ED or neighborhood.[14] This point was a valuable one in reminding the council of the value of telemedicine to create equality of care.

Dr. Randolph explained that he was open to changes in his model, but he also needed their cooperation to avoid too much complexity. Recognizing that he could not provide four different models in addition to the one he already had in place, he requested some consensus from the CEOs. After the second meeting, Dr. Randolph met with the CEO of the StESH North Campus for guidance. This CEO offered to work with Dr. Randolph as his champion on the council and had his staff pull EMS data from across the system to show where the system was losing patients to other providers or patients were traveling long distances to get acute care. With these data, Dr. Randolph and the North CEO were better able to navigate the competing interests of the various facilities.

After working together, they ultimately convinced the entire council that every facility had needs that could be met with improved acute teleneurology services. From here, they recognized that the two smaller hospitals actually needed 24/7 ER coverage and offered a plan to those CEOs that allowed them to keep their current neurologists happy by removing them from acute call responsibilities but keeping them for daytime responsibilities. For the two larger facilities, they found that a cooperative plan to bring both to comprehensive stroke status would require shared resources, and these two hospital CEOs formed a close working relationship to champion teleneurology at their facilities as part of a broader mission to become centers of excellence for neurosciences.

Takeaways

As a system of care grows, it is important to consider any strategy in the context of a needs assessment. A needs assessment is a process of questioning, collecting data, planning, and staying neutral while considering different solutions. Resources for learning more about a needs assessment are included in the reference section at the end of this chapter.

One of the most important aspects of a needs assessment is to collect data and agree on metrics. Often the research involved in data collection clarifies whether a plan is truly needed or not. It can also dispel anecdotal claims and provide a template for everyone in the system to speak the same language.

Once again, it is important not to lose track of the core value of putting the patient's needs first. While no health care system would ever claim to put profitability ahead of patient care, the business minded administrator may simply see profitability as a surrogate for doing a good job. Refocusing on metrics that capture patient care, such as "percent of stroke patients receiving tPA" or "patients treated locally without transfer," is more appropriate for growing an acute care program than simply dollars in and dollars out. In addition, in the long term, patients recognize such high-quality care and look to these kinds of hospitals for lifelong care.

The other core principle of cooperative growth is often the crux of the issue for systems. Some systems are simply more cooperative than others, while some systems see themselves as friendly rivals. In general, the needs of a hospital are always in flux, so while at a given time a facility may not see the purpose of a new service, it may in time, as coverage gaps arise, budgets shrink, call pay becomes less appealing, and competitors offer similar services.

In general, finding cooperation in a system of hospitals requires patience, seeking out a few strong allies to help with resistance, and being flexible with data-driven plans.

Summary

In this chapter, we defined the core principles of cooperative growth and serving as a fiduciary to patients. In case examples, we saw how even well-meaning, hardworking teams can be misguided as they try to grow a systems of care for telemedicine. Common pitfalls, such as forgetting stakeholders, ignoring burnout, and not recognizing variation in needs, were considered in light of the core principles, and ways forward through further education in change management, managing burnout, and conducting a needs assessment were recommended.

Many of these topics are familiar to business program graduates and hospital administrators but are rarely part of a medical school curriculum and may be a gap in a medical director's training. Adopting such skills, among others, is often necessary to build a program in a complex system of care.

References

1. Brand SL, Coon JT, Fleming LE, Carroll L, Bethel A, Wyatt K. Whole-system approaches to improving the health and wellbeing of healthcare workers: a systematic review. *PLoS ONE.* 2017;12(12). https://doi.org/10.1371/journal.pone.0188418, e0188418.
2. Broens THF, Huis in't Veld RMHA, Vollenbroek-Hutten MMR, Hermens HJ, van Halteren AT, Nieuwenhuis LJM. Determinants of successful telemedicine implementations: a literature study. *J Telemed Telecare.* 2007;13(6):303–309. https://doi.org/10.1258/135763307781644951.
3. Choi WS, Park J, Choi JYB, Yang JS. Stakeholders' resistance to telemedicine with focus on physicians: utilizing the Delphi technique. *J Telemed Telecare.* 2019;25(6):378–385. https://doi.org/10.1177/1357633X18775853.
4. Kash BA, Spaulding A, Johnson CE, Gamm L. Success factors for strategic change initiatives: a qualitative study of healthcare administrators' perspectives. *J Healthc Manag.* 2014;59(1):65–81. https://doi.org/10.1097/00115514-201401000-00011.
5. Fanale CV, Demaerschalk BM. Telestroke network business model strategies. *J Stroke Cerebrovasc Dis.* 2012;21(7):530–534. https://doi.org/10.1016/j.jstrokecerebrovasdis.2012.06.013.

6. Shanafelt TD, Noseworthy JH. Executive leadership and physician well-being: nine organizational strategies to promote engagement and reduce burnout. *Mayo Clin Proc.* 2017;92(1):129–146. https://doi.org/10.1016/j.mayocp.2016.10.004.

7. Shanafelt T, Goh J, Sinsky C. The business case for investing in physician well-being. *JAMA Intern Med.* 2017;177(12):1826–1832. https://doi.org/10.1001/jamainternmed.2017.4340.

8. Hall LH, Johnson J, Watt I, Tsipa A, O'Connor DB. Healthcare staff wellbeing, burnout, and patient safety: a systematic review. *PLoS ONE.* 2016;11(7). https://doi.org/10.1371/journal.pone.0159015, e0159015.

9. Bernard R, Cohen S. *Physician Wellness: The Rock Star Doctor's Guide: Change Your Thinking, Improve Your Life.* Rock Star Medicine Press; 2018. Retrieved from https://www.amazon.com/Physician-Wellness-Doctors-Thinking-Improve/dp/0996450939/ref=sr_1_5?dchild=1&keywords=physician+burnout&qid=1600648514&sr=8-5. Accessed 20 September 2020.

10. Ward A. *Lean Design in Healthcare: A Journey to Improve Quality and Process of Care.* Routledge; 2019. Retrieved from https://www.amazon.com/Lean-Design-Healthcare-Journey-Improve/dp/1138498793/ref=sr_1_8?dchild=1&keywords=change+management+in+healthcare&qid=1600648589&sr=8-8. Accessed 20 September 2020.

11. Doolittle GC, Spaulding RJ. Defining the needs of a telemedicine service. *J Telemed Telecare.* 2006;12(6):276–284. https://doi.org/10.1258/135763306778558150.

12. AlDossary S, Martin-Khan MG, Bradford NK, Armfield NR, Smith AC. The development of a telemedicine planning framework based on needs assessment. *J Med Syst.* 2017;41(5):1–9. https://doi.org/10.1007/s10916-017-0709-4.

13. Oest SER, Swanson MB, Ahmed A, Mohr NM. Perceptions and perceived utility of rural emergency department telemedicine services: a needs assessment. *Telemed J E-Health.* 2020;26(7):855–864. https://doi.org/10.1089/tmj.2019.0168.

14. Tatlisumak T, Soinila S, Kaste M. Telestroke networking offers multiple benefits beyond thrombolysis. *Cerebrovasc Dis.* 2009;27(4):21–27. https://doi.org/10.1159/000213055.

CHAPTER 15

Teleneurology in academics

Jillian Heisler, MD, PhD[a], Rajan Gadhia, MD[b]

[a]Physician, Neurology, Houston Methodist Hospital, Houston, TX, United States
[b]Vascular Neurologist, Neurology, Houston Methodist Hospital, Houston, TX, United States

Introduction to virtual care within graduate medical education

Virtual platforms as a means for graduate medical education have existed for many years prior to the forced use during the COVID-19 pandemic. Many programs allowed for live two-way audio-visual software for academic conferences, particularly in those programs were trainees rotate in multiple clinical settings. In fact, a number of primary care and specialty affiliate organizations at a national and international level provided some guidance on use of virtual means for conducting clinical care, albeit brief and sparsely in use. Some specialties that heavily rely on such platforms for clinical care, teaching, and research, such as vascular neurology, dermatology, and pathology were well prepared for a rapid transition to fully virtual environments in the face of the recent pandemic. Although virtual care has its limitations, its utility has been highlighted during one of the most economically burdensome pandemics to allow for continued education at all levels, and particularly in the training of residents, fellows, and medical students.

Trainee perspective on telemedicine

At the start of the COVID-19 pandemic, residency programs had to adapt quickly to ensure safety of both trainees and patients, while maintaining the academic integrity of their programs. Fortunately, many academic institutions already have the infrastructure in place for telestroke programs, making a transition in trainee clinical, academic, and research practice to virtual platforms relatively smooth. Some programs had already begun to incorporate exposure to telemedicine into their training prior to the pandemic, as this is an ever-growing method of delivering timely and effective stroke care.[1] The expansion to other areas of neurology, outside of stroke, has been an exciting, albeit challenging, byproduct of the COVID-19 pandemic, and formal incorporation into neurology residency training appears to be the natural progression in neurology and across all fields of medicine.

Teaching faculty perspective on telemedicine

Many faculty and staff members involved in training medical students, residents, and fellows were likely trained in an era where emphasis was placed on in-person teaching. In fact, this can be highlighted by the reluctance in many providers over the past decade as the transition from paper records was made to the electronic health record (EHR). Most large institutions, where many of the graduate medical programs are primarily based, made the tough and expensive decision to comply with new Centers for Medicare & Medicaid Services (CMS) recommendations for enhancing the ability to exchange health information through the implementation of some form of an EHR platform. Of course, there were many providers who felt that the EHR would truly enhance patient care through ease of electronic exchange and communication among multiple providers, care coordination and patient engagement, and for purposes of billing of patient encounters. EHR allowed for electronic attestations and review of house-staff order entry and vital signs, all from a remote location in the hopes of enhancing patient safety and clinical care.

During the early days of the uptick of coronavirus cases across the continental United States, most program directors and teaching faculty faced the exhaustive challenge of maintaining the standard of education provided to trainees in a novel and innovative way. The major benefit, and likely impetus for doing so, was the early shortage of necessary personal protective equipment for providers, the insufficient testing at the time, and the need to protect trainees from a disease that we knew very little about. Almost overnight, recommendations and guidance were provided by the different academies within specialties regarding the use of virtual care to provide clinical care, conduct research, and continue to provide educational lectures and experiences to students. Cohorts of trainees were reassigned roles, education and resources were provided on conducting visits virtually, and social distancing measures were enforced in all clinical and nonclinical settings. Instead of in-person morning report or noon conference lectures, virtual teleconferencing platforms such as Zoom, WebEx, Microsoft Teams, and many others were implemented and utilized to continue the trainee experience. Program directors and faculty members who were well versed in utilizing technology were given the additional task of training other less experienced faculty and staff on the workings of these platforms for clinical care, academics, research, and administrative tasks. The Accreditation Council for Graduate Medical Education (ACGME) began to prepare and provide further guidance on the recommendations for training programs on continued education.

Surveys and other feedback mechanisms were put forth by the ACGME to track the modifications to trainee experience during the months of the COVID-19 pandemic. In fact, in order to continue in some fashion a normal academic year timeline, typically unimaginable in-person events were transitioned to be conducted virtually, including graduation ceremonies and house-staff and faculty social gatherings and retreats.

Clinical

Clinical duties in residency fall under two broad categories, inpatient and ambulatory, although inpatient time is heavily favored in most training programs, particularly in the early years of training. At the onset of the pandemic, there was a significant amount of uncertainty regarding how to continue clinical practice in both settings while ensuring the safety of trainees and patients. At institutions that rely on the resident workforce, it is of paramount importance to keep residents safe and healthy to maintain adequate staffing. Virtual medicine is just one avenue of many that has been embraced in both settings to allow for safe delivery of patient care.

Residents are often on the frontlines of patient care in the inpatient setting. Neurology residents are frequently called on to evaluate patients emergently in both the emergency room and on the wards, for the assessment of a variety of acute neurologic conditions including stroke, seizure, and encephalopathy. While initially perceived as more challenging than ambulatory care, inpatient virtual care has been rapidly adapted to effectively care for patients at all levels of acuity and in a variety of inpatient clinical settings, although prior to the pandemic, there was only sparse utilization of acute inpatient virtual care means for patient care by trainees. During the COVID-19 surges, those responsible for training programs were forced to map out innovative ways to continue to care for patients, while keeping trainees and faculty safe, but at the same time preventing unnecessary use of a limited resource of personal protective equipment.

In a hub-and-spoke model of stroke care, spoke hospitals have access to neurologists via telemedicine platforms. At a typical comprehensive stroke center, namely in an academic setting staffed by residents, patients are evaluated face-to-face, and in most instances there was no previous need for telemedicine. Neurology residents may be the first point of contact in the evaluation of acute stroke patients, and often complete their assessment and give a verbal report to an attending faculty member by phone in order to make joint treatment decisions. In the midst of a pandemic, this has the potential to expose residents unknowingly to highly infectious patients, even with appropriate screening processes in place. Utilization of telemedicine has the potential to reduce these exposures significantly, while allowing for timely assessment of acute stroke patients. "Code stroke" pathways have been rapidly modified to include the use of telemedicine following emergency guidelines from the American Stroke Association,[2] and have proven to be effective methods in protecting both health care providers and patients.[3,4] Being the first line in the care of acute stroke patients can be a significant source of anxiety for young residents, who are expected to assess these patients accurately in order to make rapid treatment decisions in an ever-changing field. Adding the risk of infection with COVID-19, this can be a daunting task, particularly for residents who are inexperienced in managing acute patients in any setting. With the introduction of telemedicine platforms into residency training, attending faculty members can supervise the virtual assessment of patients in real-time alongside residents if needed. This provides an additional safety net for residents who may be uncertain of their diagnostic abilities, and allows for rapid feedback, instruction, and guidance on treatment decisions from their supervising attending.

The classic model of academic hospital rounds led by an attending faculty, with a large group of residents and trainees and other disciplines, has also required a paradigm shift. Due to social distancing protocols, minimizing the number of team members during rounds attempts to limit nosocomial and intra-team transmission throughout the hospital. Effective and safe rounds can largely be accomplished virtually, using a variety of platforms to perform virtual "table rounds," virtual assessments of patients, and communicate plans of care among team members. From the resident perspective, virtual rounds can save a substantial amount of time in some respects, by reducing the amount of time dedicated to in-person rounds throughout the hospital. Virtual table rounds may also offer additional teaching opportunities, including review of pertinent laboratory and imaging findings on personal devices while maintaining social distancing measures. Physical assessment of patients can be accomplished with designated video-capable tablets or other handheld devices with the assistance of a family member or bedside nurse, and with the device adequately disinfected between patients. This limits not only the exposure of the health care provider to patients, but also the exposure of the patients to multiple teams of health care providers. In an intensive care unit (ICU) setting that is equipped with virtual ICU technology, this can be utilized to communicate with the alert patient or for observation of the nonalert patient with the assistance of the bedside nurse for some exam maneuvers. The major benefit of many of these platforms is the ability to allow third-party members, particularly family members, to see loved ones while restricted visitor access policies are in place during the pandemic. It allows for real time monitoring of vital signs, medication administration, intravenous drips, and frequent clinical assessments.

In the ambulatory care setting, many virtual platforms allow multiple users to participate in video calls, and thus both trainee and attending faculty can simultaneously participate in the evaluation of patients. The resident can take on the primary role of obtaining pertinent history and performing a virtual exam, under the direct supervision of an attending. This provides additional educational guidance and opportunities for one-on-one instruction, which is especially useful in mastering the teleneurology physical exam. It also allows for additional guidance and molding of the trainee's history taking ability, which is often not directly supervised by teaching faculty. The use of telemedicine in the ambulatory care setting has also extended the possibility of residents working from home. Those residents on ambulatory rotations can participate in virtual clinics, and thus create a pool of residents who are reserved for backup of essential rotations in the event that staffing becomes compromised by illness. Attending faculty members also reevaluated staffing models to allow for less frequent rotation and extended blocks of time on and off service in order to allow for an alternative backup pool in the event that one may become infected and require quarantine.

Prior to the COVID-19 pandemic, many residents and attending faculty had only a cursory exposure to virtual care visits, if any exposure at all, as virtual visits have not been a significant part of typical ambulatory care. This has become an increasingly valuable part of clinical practice education and teaching, with a rapid and steep learning curve for both trainees and faculty. It has become fairly clear that teleneurology and telemedicine will be a consistent part of clinical practice now and in the future. From the viewpoint of faculty members, if residents are exposed to virtual ambulatory care at regular intervals and as an integrated part of their training, the next generation of practicing physicians will be well equipped to implement telemedicine in their routine clinical practice. Additional competencies are likely to be added to the current clinical milestone criteria for demonstrating clearance for independent practice without supervision.

Academics

A substantial amount of time during residency is dedicated to didactic teaching on the part of the faculty, and learning on the side of the trainee, outside of clinical practice. This takes a variety of different forms including lecture presentations from faculty, case conferences with residents and supervising faculty, preparation of and delivering talks on areas of progress within neurology by residents, attending meetings on special areas of interest, preparation for the board exam, and even participating in medical student education. Frequently this involves residents, faculty members and other trainees gathering in close quarters.

Limitations on the number of individuals allowed to meet in person has resulted in the expanded use of teleconferencing platforms in medical education. While there are occasional technical drawbacks like poor internet connectivity, by and large the transition to primarily web-based didactic sessions was a smooth process. Benefits to web-based conferences include accessibility—residents can participate in conferences via tablet, smartphone, or computer from any location, which can allow residents to work from home when they are on nonessential or elective rotations. Many programs have trainees and faculty that rotate at multiple facilities and who may not be on site to attend in-person educational conferences, for which a virtual conference medium has led to increased participation. Likewise, speakers from outside institutions may be more easily accessible without need for travel, opening avenues for exposure to areas of expertise that may not be well represented at the home institution. In 2020, the American Academy of Neurology (AAN) also made accessible the materials and lectures for the annual meeting, and provided all members, including trainees, with free access. This allowed some residents and faculty members who have never had the opportunity to attend this meeting with access to valuable educational materials that may not have been readily available during previous years.

Despite the ease of use and possible benefit of increased accessibility, there are a number of limitations to be considered when implementing web-based learning as a substitution for face-to-face conferences. In the in-person learning environment, resident participation and engagement are frequently better than via teleconference. In fact, faculty participation and engagement also has the potential to be more passive. Active participation with the speaker and immediate feedback from residents can be a struggle when conducting meetings via web-based services, as it is easier for residents to continue with multitasking when hidden behind a screen. Residents may also experience "screen fatigue," as a large part of the workday is spent in front of a screen for review of patient information, video visits, and didactic learning. In the future, a combination of in-person and virtual learning may be able to strike a balance between the benefits and limitations of web-based conferences. Furthermore, while the AAN has the ability as a large organization to provide conference materials at low cost, smaller organizations and meetings may not be capable of such broad access, and thus residents with interest in subspecialty conferences may be at a disadvantage if the restrictions of 2020 continue.

Research

In some ways, research in residency may be the simplest activity to convert to a solely virtual practice, particularly retrospective studies with chart review. Most case scenarios, in fact, are already conducted electronically with review of imaging and the EHR, and in some cases remotely. Unless participating in basic science bench research or clinical trials that require active treatment and evaluation of patients, most research activities that residents participate in require individual efforts of composing a clinical question, chart review, literature review, and write-up. Collaboration with colleagues and advising faculty can be achieved via teleconference or videoconference. The COVID-19 pandemic has also offered a unique opportunity for research across many disciplines, with the possibility of rapid acquisition of data due to the influx of cases and expedited processes for publication. Research and pursuit of publication is a valuable process for residents to be actively involved in to hone critical thinking and communication skills.

The ability to communicate and interpret research and scientific data effectively is an invaluable skill, particularly with respect to public speaking. Presentation of research at conferences, whether local, national, or international, is one of the primary methods by which residents gain experience in this skill. The most accessible mode of presentation is through poster sessions, in which residents can practice their communication skills in a smaller group setting and often one-on-one. Unfortunately, this method of presentation is not readily adaptable to teleconferencing platforms. Speaking engagements, including grand rounds presentations, are more easily transitioned to virtual platforms, and are perhaps a slightly less daunting task when performed virtually versus in-person. Whether through their home programs or in conference settings, residents should be encouraged to participate in such speaking engagements, and they may be more willing in the setting of a virtual platform as some of the pressure of speaking to a large audience is relieved when that audience is primarily out of sight.

Research in the sense of large randomized clinical trials poses yet another challenge during the pandemic. Many studies halted enrollment during peak surges to prevent exposure of faculty and staff, and due to limitation in resources, and study materials. In the broad sense, however, the COVID-19 era has brought forward decades of advancement in clinical, translational, and basic science research with the means of expanding enrollment and inclusion with virtual platforms. Use of electronic signature for electronic consenting, performing physical exams virtually for the purpose of assessing inclusion and exclusion criteria, and involvement of family members through multiparty conferences for consenting by proxy in certain situations have all been made possible due to rapid adaption to technology. As a result, many of the clinical trials that were halted at the beginning of the pandemic were able to continue their enrollment with the rollout of a virtual consenting and enrollment process.

Administrative

The transition and rapid expansion of telemedicine and virtual education requires coordination of efforts among faculty members, residents, and ancillary staff. Prior to the COVID-19 pandemic, many individuals had little or no exposure to the now commonly used and widely embraced virtual platforms. Transition to virtual care is a steep learning curve for some, and adequate technical support is necessary to make the transition as smooth as possible. As there was quick realization, many departments recognized "champions," or leaders who could assist in the training, education, and rollout of virtual platforms. Faculty and trainees equally required guidance, and a robust infrastructure in information technology was created to help meet the demand required to assess and use case scenarios specific to individual practices and practitioners, address bandwidth, and remain available for troubleshooting.

During a time of rapid change, there is also a need to disseminate the most up-to-date information quickly to a wide range of clinical staff. This has required a transition to web-based platforms to hold large meetings, both system-wide and departmental. Frequent administrative faculty meetings, which are typically conducted in-person, were quickly transitioned to virtual platforms to abide by social distancing measures. Additionally, town halls and resident rotation feedback sessions can and were conducted virtually to allow for ongoing program director and trainee feedback. A unique challenge that will take place in the first interview season after the outbreak of COVID-19 is the need to conduct recruitment and a match virtually. This requires use of a virtual platform and extensive scheduling to ensure that a "room-to-room" workflow, albeit virtual, remains on an interview day. Marketing of a program becomes difficult due to the inability for trainees out of state or city to visualize themselves in the environment that they may spend the next few years training. Institutional GME programs have offered to make video walk-throughs of the hospital and clinic settings, and to assist in creating a proper interview day experience as good as possible. It remains to be seen how the first cycle of matching training programs will adjust to the new normal, for now.

Final thoughts from trainee and mentee

In some ways, the COVID-19 pandemic brought us into the future of medicine by accelerating and expanding the use of virtual care throughout all aspects of medicine. From expanded clinical use in both the inpatient and ambulatory care settings, to teaching and instruction of residents and medical students, virtual platforms have proven to be effective methods of delivering care and education. We propose that, moving forward, some form of a hybrid of in-person and virtual means will exist in the continued education of future trainees.

References

1. Tipton PW, D'Souza CE, Greenway MRF, et al. Incorporation of telestroke into neurology residency training: "time is brain and education". *Telemed J E Health.* 2019;26(8):1035–1042. https://doi.org/10.1089/tmj.2019.0184.
2. AHA/ASA Stroke Council Leadership. Temporary emergency guidance to US stroke centers during the coronavirus disease 2019 (COVID-19) pandemic: on behalf of the American Heart Association/American Stroke Association stroke council leadership. *Stroke.* 2020;51:1910–1912. https://doi.org/10.1161/STROKEAHA.120.030023.
3. Meyer D, Meyer BC, Rapp KS, et al. A stroke care model at an academic, comprehensive stroke center during the 2020 COVID-19 pandemic. *J Stroke Cerebrovasc Dis.* 2020;29(8). https://doi.org/10.1016/j.jstrokecerebrovasdis.2020.104927, 104927.
4. Heisler JM, Etherton MR, Viswanathan A, Schwamm L, Gadhia RR. COVID-care: rapid expansion of an existing telestroke infrastructure to battle a pandemic. *Int J Neurol Dis.* 2020;4(1):038–041.

CHAPTER 16

Telehealth laws, regulations, and reimbursement

George Williams, MD, FASA, FCCM, FCCP[a,b]**, Randall Wright, MD**[c,d]

[a]Medical Co-Director, LBJ Surgical Intensive Care Unit, Houston, TX, United States
[b]Vice Chair for Critical Care Medicine, UT Houston Department of Anesthesiology, Houston, TX, United States
[c]Director of the Brain Wellness and Sleep Program, Houston Methodist Hospital, The Woodlands, TX, United States
[d]Clinical Faculty EnMed, Texas A&M University College of Medicine, College of Engineering, Houston, TX, United States

Introduction

The legal, regulatory, and reimbursement aspects of incorporating telehealth into a neurological practice are likely the aspects of this technology that have been the source of the most trepidation for neurologist and other practitioners. The novelty of this modality of practice has led to an ever-changing legal landscape over recent years. Prior to March 6, 2020, one may argue that progress being made in creating a more favorable regulatory landscape for telemedicine in the United States was slower than many of us would have hoped for. However, the world changed in March 2020 with several sentinel events that started a chain reaction that profoundly ushered telemedicine onto center stage. On that day, President Trump closed the US borders to international travel, the NBA abruptly canceled its season and any games that were being played at the time, and Tom Hanks revealed that he was infected with COVID-19 and was in self-quarantine; the citizens of the United States of America realized that COVID-19 was becoming a crisis on US soil.

In the days that followed, the US underwent an unprecedented national shutdown of all nonessential businesses and, in an instant, all of the country's nonemergent medical practices came to a screeching halt. When the age-old art of patient care seemed to enter one of its darkest moments, the savior was the budding technology of telemedicine. The days that followed produced an unprecedented flurry of regulatory changes that released the genie of telemedicine out of its restrictive bottle and allowed it to prop up the medical community during its most critical time. The ensuing days and weeks showed regulation after regulation and state after state passing laws that allowed physicians across the United States to practice telemedicine without the shackles that had bound them previously. For the first time, millions of patients and doctors established relationships virtually and were able to continue and initiate care from the safety of their homes.

By the time you read this book, we are confident that the laws will have changed as the COVID-19 pandemic continues to evolve and the appetite of the world grows for convenient care from the comfort of home. For this reason, writing a chapter on the laws, regulations, and reimbursement opportunities for your practice is a nearly impossible task, but a necessary one. The laws that govern your practice in your state at the time you are trying to implement telemedicine into your practice will be very different from where they are at the time this book goes into print. Therefore, our approach will be to provide a framework for you to understand the concepts at play that govern our practice of telehealth and provide you with the resources to navigate the undulating waters of telehealth regulation.

To start the journey in the regulation of telehealth, we must first start to define a few terms and concepts. In regards to what telemedicine is, one may look at it as a modality through which one may practice medicine rather than a subspecialty of a medical practice. The technology through which one may practice telemedicine is ever evolving. The American Telemedicine Association refers to the different modalities of telehealth delivery as services. They, along with many other institutions, define four basic services or modalities of telehealth delivery (Fig. 16.1)[1]:

- **Live Videoconferencing or Real Time Audio-Video Communication (Synchronous)**
  This is the traditional model of delivering telehealth services that most people think of and is the model for which many of the initial laws on telehealth are written. This is when a practitioner and a patient communicate in real time using a secure means of video/audio communication. The communication may also be between two health care professionals.
- **Store and Forward (Asynchronous)**
  This modality of health care utilizes nonreal time ways for a practitioner and a patient to communicate. It utilizes the storage of medical information (images, vital signs, electroencephalography (EEG) data, etc.) and the subsequent transmission of that data for the review by a practitioner at a later time. This may be an important area in the future, as it allows patients to upload information, and the doctor to review and make decisions, both in their own time.
- **Remote Patient Monitoring (RPM)**
  This modality of health care involves the use of devices to remotely collect medical data from patients in their homes or other nonmedical

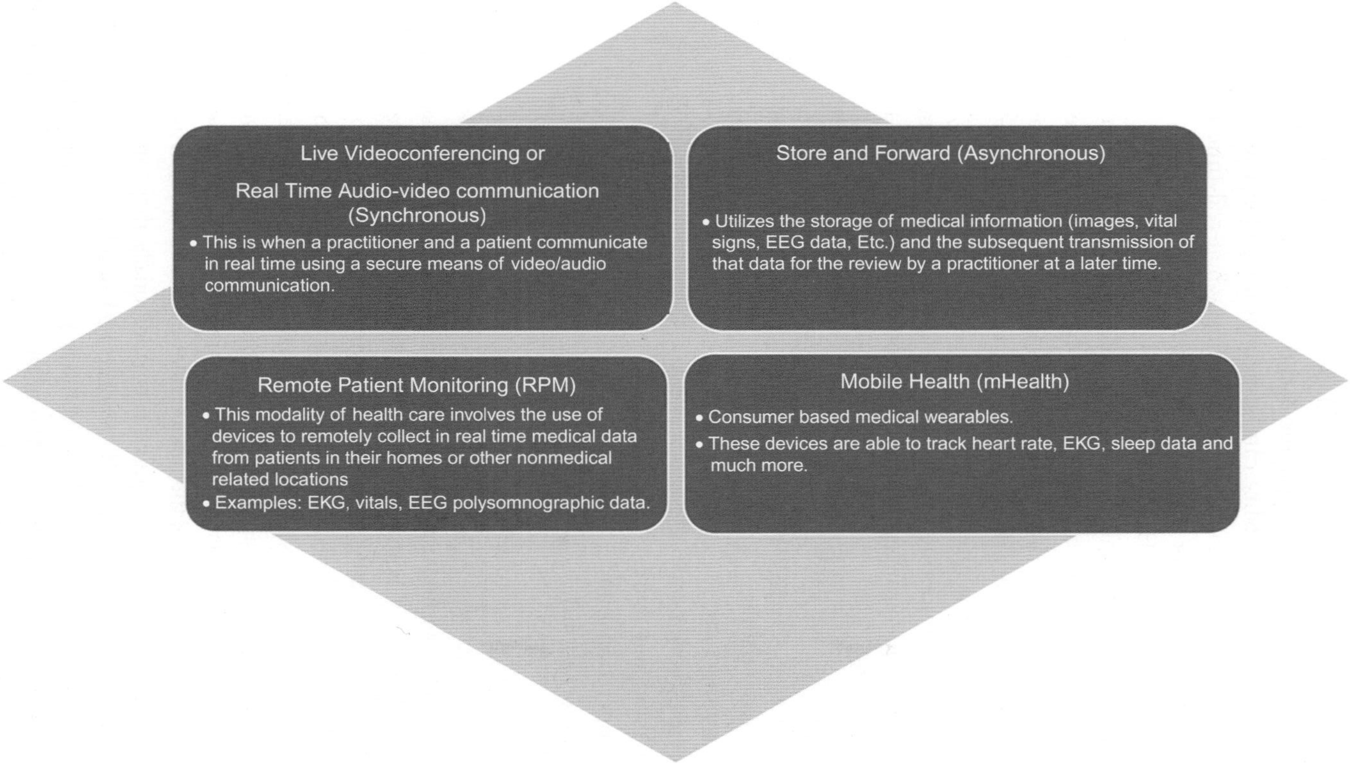

Live Videoconferencing or Real Time Audio-video communication (Synchronous)
- This is when a practitioner and a patient communicate in real time using a secure means of video/audio communication.

Store and Forward (Asynchronous)
- Utilizes the storage of medical information (images, vital signs, EEG data, Etc.) and the subsequent transmission of that data for the review by a practitioner at a later time.

Remote Patient Monitoring (RPM)
- This modality of health care involves the use of devices to remotely collect in real time medical data from patients in their homes or other nonmedical related locations
- Examples: EKG, vitals, EEG polysomnographic data.

Mobile Health (mHealth)
- Consumer based medical wearables.
- These devices are able to track heart rate, EKG, sleep data and much more.

Fig. 16.1 Four basic services or modalities of telehealth delivery.[1]

related locations and transmit that data to a central location for evaluation. Such information my include electrocardiogram (EKG), vitals, EEG, or even polysomnographic data that could be monitored remotely in real time. This modality can be helpful for patients who are housebound, or even during diagnostic testing when real-time information could be lifesaving or prevent hospitalization.

- **Mobile Health (mHealth)**
  This refers to the exploding industry of consumer-based medical wearables. These devices are able to track heart rate, EKG, sleep data, and much more. Many direct-to-consumer companies are engaging in this tech space and we will be seeing more companies and devices come to the market in the future.

When considering incorporating telehealth into your practice, there are several medical/legal topics you should consider, which include:
1. licensure;
2. practice standards;
3. privacy and security;
4. credentialing;
5. contracting;
6. reimbursement;
7. fraud and abuse;
8. operational; and
9. international.

Licensure

The first step in starting using telemedicine in your practice is to make sure you understand licensing. Fortunately, the rules regarding this topic are well established and relatively straightforward. A doctor must be licensed in the state in which the patient is located at the time of the telehealth consult. So, if you wish to see a patient from Louisiana, you need to have a Louisiana license. However, if you plan to see patients from different states, the rules are such that you will need to have a license in each state in which you are planning to see patients and you will also need to be aware of the unique rules each state has, such as Continuing Medical Education (CME) requirements. Additionally, there are four types of licensure through which a state may regulate a telehealth practice.

The first is full licensure, which would require a physician or other health professional to obtain an unrestricted license. The second is a recognition of licensure policy, in which one state may "recognize" the license of another state. This would be facilitated by an endorsement, mutual recognition, or reciprocity agreement. Endorsement permits a state medical board to issue a license to a physician from another state when equivalent licensing standards are in place. Mutual recognition permits a state medical board simply to accept the licensure policies of the physician's home state. A reciprocity agreement allows a physician in one state to have equal privileges in another state without being required to register for a separate license. The third is a consultation exception. This is an older mechanism in several states, which allows physicians from outside states to consult occasionally with patients within the state in question without obtaining an additional license. This is usually applicable when a physician licensed by the state of the patient has primary responsibility to care for that patient. The fourth type is special licensure, which was promoted by the Federation of State Medical Boards starting in 1996 and has been adopted by 22 states thus far. This proposal is now known as the Interstate Medical Licensure Compact and is very similar in concept to the second type of licensure approach discussed above. More information about this can be found at www.imlcc.org. This approach requires special licensure procedures for physicians practicing telemedicine across state lines, and at the same time preserves the current state licensure systems. The fifth model would be national licensure, which currently does not exist in the US for private practice. An existing system analogous to national licensure would be physicians practicing telemedicine in the Armed Forces or the Veterans Affairs hospital system.

These systems have multiple nuances, so it is important to consult your health care attorney to review your specific needs before starting your new multistate telemedicine program.

Practice standards

The concept of practice standards exists on a state-by-state basis. They are governed by your state medical boards and typically can be reviewed on a state medical board's website. Many states have a telemedicine section and should list any practice standards that may exist. Each state has different standards, so this will be required reading for you prior to you initiating your telehealth practice. Many of the rules are not very complicated, but you need to be aware of the ones that govern the states in which you plan to practice. There is tremendous variety in the propensity for disciplinary action based on each state's medical boards and their norms. For example, Delaware has the highest amount (10.27) of yearly disciplinary actions rate

Table 16.1 Common topics related to standards of practice.

Informed telemedicine consent
New vs. established patients
Verification of patient identity
Restrictions on site of origination
Use of a patient-site telepresenter
Modality of communication
Remote prescribing
Record keeping
Record sharing
Patient choice of provider
Disclosures
Malpractice insurance
Credentialing

per 1000 physicians compared to the District of Columbia, which has the lowest (1.74). A variety of topics are covered in the practice standards, and a few common ones are listed in Table 16.1.

Payment

The landscape of payment for medical services, like the regulatory laws that govern its activities, is shifting. New models are being tested and introduced all over the country and the rise of telemedicine is injecting itself into the middle of it. So, when thinking about getting compensated for your tele-medicine services, payment from the government or insurer may not be your only option. Of note, the term "reimbursement" is commonly used, but has the unintended consequence of implying that the physician has "money to burn" and can wait to get paid back. Using the term "payment" is most accurate because you are being appropriately compensated for a service provided. A few examples of ways in which providers may receive payment for their services are: governmental payers (Medicare, Medicaid), commercial insurance plans, consumer cost saving plans, consumer cost sharing plans (Medishare), contracted institutional contracts, and business service agreements.

Medicare

Medicare, prior to the COVID-19 crisis, was rather limiting on the param-eters for which it would reimburse for teleservices. Prior to COVID-19, Medicare would reimburse for teleservices according to the Social Security

Act of 1835(m) or 42 USC 1395 m. Such limitations required the patient to be located at one of eight qualifying facilities (originating site) in a qualifying rural area. Services could only be provided by one of 10 eligible professionals and the technology had to be a real-time audio-video connection. However, as of March 6, 2020, Medicare expanded its coverage of telehealth services due to the COVID-19 public health emergency. From that date, doctors and other health providers could use telehealth means to treat COVID-19 patients and other medically reasonable conditions and receive payment. The geographic locations of the patients were expanded to include offices, hospitals, and places of residence.[2] This change opened the door for providers to start caring for patients virtually and allowed millions of patients to seek the care they desperately needed during a time when leaving the home was perceived as a potential hazard. This expansion of benefits was done on a temporary and emergency basis under the 1135 waiver authority and the Coronavirus Preparedness and Response Supplemental Appropriations Act.[3]

The expansion of telehealth services includes three areas of telehealth services: telehealth visits, virtual check-ins, and e-visits (Fig. 16.2). The act also allowed (subject to state laws) payment to physicians, nurse practitioners, physician assistants, nurse midwives, certified nurse anesthetists, clinical psychologists, clinical social workers, registered dietitians, and nutrition professionals for the covered telehealth services. At that time, only established patients were covered, but Health and Human Services (HHS) did announce that "To the extent the 1135 waiver requires an established relationship, HHS will not conduct audits to ensure that such a prior relationship existed for claims submitted during this public health emergency."

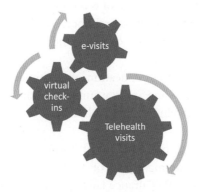

Fig. 16.2 Medicare 2020 COVID-19 expansion of telehealth services.

Earlier in this chapter, we defined four basic types of telehealth services (real time audio-visual, store and forward, remote patient monitoring, and mobile health). The practical implications of these general modalities are mentioned in the Medicare coverage of specifically mentioned modalities: telehealth visits, virtual check-ins, and e-visits.

The telehealth visits are defined as the traditionally structured interactive audio and video interaction between and provider and a patient in real time. Virtual check-ins are a little different. They are defined as brief communications between provider and patient. The patient must consent verbally to this type of encounter. This service is a patient-initiated synchronous discussion with the provider via a number of communication modalities. The practitioner can respond to the patient's request via telephone Healthcare Common Procedure Coding System (HCPCS) (code G2012), audio/video, secure text, email, or the now popular use of a patient portal. These virtual check-ins are reported to be approved for reimbursement with the intention of giving patients a technology-based means of communicating with their doctors to help avoid unnecessary trips to the doctor's office. These check-ins are for established/existing patients where the communication is not related to an office visit within the prior seven days and does not lead to a medical visit within the next 24 h or next available appointment. In addition to the virtual check-ins, patients can also send their physician captured video (or HCPCS code G2010).[4]

The final visit type is e-visits. With this modality, established Medicare patients who also give verbal consent may initiate a nonface-to-face communication with their doctor through their online patient portal. For these visits, the patient must initiate the communication and it can occur over a 7-day time frame. CPT codes 99421-99423 and HCPCS codes G2061-G2063 can be used as applicable.

One final modality to be aware of is remote patient monitoring (RPM). There are many nuances to getting reimbursed, but Medicare does provide reimbursement for modality. As of 2019, the new CPT codes for RPM were as follows:

- 99453—setup and patient education of equipment use.
- 99454—device recording and transmission each 30 days.
- 99457—20 min of clinical staff, physician, or other qualified health professional.

The state level laws on commercial coverage of medical services are another constantly changing aspect of medical payment. Most states have some form of commercial insurance law regarding telehealth. Each state has different laws requiring insurance companies to cover telehealth services.

However, a law simply requiring an insurance company to cover telehealth services is not the end of the story. Payment parity laws are also needed to ensure that amount reimbursed for telehealth visits is reimbursed at a rate equivalent to an in-person visit.

Venturing into the telehealth space does open the door to new areas of fraud and abuse.[5] It is important to be aware of potential areas of risk when venturing into your new telemedicine practice. Prior laws on such topics are still enforced and should always be considered as you venture into you new style of practice. Areas to be aware of are listed in Table 16.2.

The role of advocacy

As telehealth is gaining a larger and larger role in the delivery of health care, advocacy groups are now beginning to form. The Taskforce on Telehealth Policy is an effort between the American Telemedicine Association, the National Committee for Quality Assurance (NCQA), and the Alliance for Connected Care in order to meet the goal of influencing telehealth policy on a national level. The goal as currently stated is to provide "consensus recommendations for policymakers on how to maximize the benefits of telehealth services while maintaining high standards for patient safety and program integrity." But who are the actual people that will write these recommendations? Is there a committee comprised of stakeholders, physicians, and organizations? What funding does this group have and how much?

As one can see, the discussion of policy and how to influence it is a significant one. It is important for you to communicate with legislators and regulators about laws that affect your practice. Without the input of their constituents, leaders cannot be expected to make good decisions for your patients. Furthermore, it is absolutely critical that you vote in every election, regardless of whether it is a local or a presidential election cycle. This is because how you vote is secret, but *if* you vote is a matter of public record. Legislative staffers commonly look up the voting records of those who call

Table 16.2 Topics to consider to avoid fraud and abuse.

Federal laws	State laws
Antikickback	Self-referral
Self-referral	Fee splitting
Civil monetary penalties	Patient brokering
	Corporate practice of medicine

Source: Ferrante TJ, Esq, Lecture entitled "Laws, regulations and compliance in telemedicine: what you need to know". Master Clinicians Winter 2019 Telemedicine Conference 2019.

or meet with them, and if the constituent that is advocating does not regularly vote, they are more likely to dismiss the content of your conversation even if the legislator was engaging and interested in your discussion.

Money also has a role in politics, and political action committees (PACs) are a way to pool funds collectively for a specific cause. These funds can be used to contribute to campaigns of candidates and even hire lobbyists. Organizations that have PACs include the American Medical Association, the American Academy of Neurology, and the American College of Physicians, to name a few. These entities serve to communicate with legislators at the state and federal level issues that are important to the practice of medicine, the practice of telehealth (when applicable), and issues that lead to better care for the patients that we take care of on a daily basis. In effect, a PAC is an IRS/Federal Election Commission-recognized bank account, which solely serves the purpose of contributing to political candidates supportive to the issues of medicine. Similarly, there are PACs for lawyers, nurses, teachers, etc., for similar purposes. Organizational dues alone are not adequate to support the functions of political advocacy for many reasons, including some tax laws. In the 2018 election cycle, $54.5 million in PAC funds pertaining to health care were collected and contributed to candidates. While there is not a PAC specifically for the purpose of telehealth known to the authors as of the production of this book, it is likely only a matter of time until one is founded.

References

1. https://www.americantelemed.org.
2. American Academy of Neurology COVID-19 Telemedicine Page n.d.
3. United States COVID-19 Emergency Declaration Health Care Providers Fact Sheet n.d.
4. Medicare. https://www.medicare.gov/coverage/telehealth.
5. Ferrante TJ. Esq, Lecture entitled "Laws, regulations and compliance in telemedicine: what you need to know". In: *Master Clinicians Winter 2019 Telemedicine Conference*; 2019.

Further reading

6. Center for Telehealth and e-Health Law n.d.
7. http://www.imlcc.org.
8. CMS Fact Sheet. https://www.cms.gov/newsroom/fact-sheets/medicare-telemedicine-health-care-provider-fact-sheet.
9. Cwiek MA, Rafiq A, Qamar A, Tobey C, Merrell RC. Telemedicine licensure in the United States: the need for a cooperative regional approach. *Telemed J E Health.* 2007;13(2):141–147. https://doi.org/10.1089/tmj.2006.0029.
10. Cwiek MA, Rafiq A, Qamar A, Tobey C, Merrell RC. Telemedicine licensure in the United States: the need for a cooperative regional approach. *Telemed J E Health.* 2007;13(2):141–147. https://doi.org/10.1089/tmj.2006.0029.

CHAPTER 17

International teleneurology

Esther Cubo, MD, PhD
Neurology Department, Hospital Universitario Burgos, University of Burgos, Burgos, Spain

Background

Traditional medical practice is not always the most efficient or convenient way to provide care to our neurology patients. With an increasing demand for neurologic services in a growing population, technology can be one way to extend our reach to our patients. As technologies develop, it is paramount that practitioners maintain high-quality care, equivalent to traditional in-person visits. Information and communication technologies (ICTs) have great potential to address some of the challenges both developed and developing countries face in providing accessible, cost-effective, and high-quality health care services. Telemedicine uses ICTs to overcome geographical barriers and increase access to health care services, and is particularly beneficial for rural and underserved communities, groups that traditionally suffer from lack of access to health care.[1] In this chapter, we will first discuss the rationale behind using teleneurology in different parts of the world including the different aspects of telemedicine such as tele-expertise (seeking the second opinion of one or more medical professionals regarding elements of the patient's medical file), teleconsultation (remote consultations with a patient), and tele-education; and secondly, we will include the most representative international examples of teleneurology initiatives.

The burden of neurological disorders

According to the World Health Organization (WHO) in collaboration with the World Federation of Neurology, there are inadequate resources for patients with neurological disorders in most parts of the world, highlighting inequalities in the access to neurological care across different populations, and in particular in those living in low-income countries and underserved regions of the world.[2] Neurological disorders are increasingly recognized as major causes of death and disability worldwide. Although age-standardized incidence, mortality, and prevalence rates of many neurological disorders declined for many countries from 1990 to 2015, the absolute number of people affected by, dying from, or remaining disabled from neurological disorders over the past 25 years has been increasing globally.[3] In the last report of the Global Burden of Diseases (GBD), Injuries, and Risk Factors Study (GBD) 2016,[4] globally, neurological disorders were the leading cause of Disability Adjusted Life Year (DALYs) (276 million [95% UI 247–308]) and the second leading cause of deaths (9.0 million [8.8–9.4]). The four largest contributors of neurological DALYs were stroke (42.2% [38.6–46.1]), migraine (16.3% [11.7–20.8]), Alzheimer's and other dementias (10.4% [9.0–12.1]), and meningitis (7.9% [6.6–10.4]). As populations are growing and aging, and the prevalence of major disabling and neurodegenerative neurological disorders steeply increases with age, governments will face increasing demand for treatment, rehabilitation, and support services for neurological disorders. The scarcity of established modifiable risks for most of the neurological burden and the shortage of neurological services demonstrate that new knowledge is required to develop effective prevention and treatment strategies, to ensure equitable access.[4] In this regard, teleneurology can be considered as an efficient and feasible alternative tool.[5]

Clinical care

International telestroke networks

Around the world, equitable access to best practice acute stroke care, including stroke thrombolysis and thrombectomy, is still a major challenge.[6] Services in low-population density or economically deprived countries may struggle to provide an expert service 24/7. To tackle the limitation of access, telemedicine for acute stroke care, otherwise known as telestroke, has been developed and implemented in several countries over the past two decades.[7] Thrombolysis via telestroke is an accepted alternative[8] and has been proven to be safe and effective.[9] In contrast, international teleradiology services have utilized telemedicine for several years,[10] and publications about the feasibility of an international telestroke network have been published in the last 10 years.[11] Telestroke networks have been successfully operated, first in the USA and Canada, followed by other regions in the world. The Telemedicine Pilot Project for Integrative Stroke Care (TEMPiS) was the first pilot teleneurology network outside the USA dedicated to stroke management, established in 2002, supported by a Bavarian state grant. TEMPiS has since transitioned to be supported by regular health insurance and is built around two comprehensive stroke centers in eastern Bavaria. The network provided 10,239 neurology consultations between February 2003 and December 2006, and about 5.8% of the ischemic stroke patients were given thrombolytic therapy during this period.[5, 12] In another international example, Ranta et al. reported the feasibility of an international telestroke service between Scotland and New Zealand taking advantage of international time zone differences. After addressing medico, legal, and technical issues, this program was found feasible, improving access to expert care in regions where stroke specialist input is limited. However, the sustainability of telestroke programs can also be an issue. These authors[13] also reported the impact of telestroke service discontinuation on service provision within a regional and national context. They found that the thrombolysis rate and door-to-needle time decreased after the pilot experience, returning to baseline services, indicating that a brief, transient implementation of a telestroke program is insufficient to upskill provincial hospital generalist clinicians.

Nowadays, the use of telestroke programs for acute care is expanding. Various models of telestroke have been used in different regions and countries.[14] To standardize the quality of these international programs, the establishment of consensus minimum dataset for acute telestroke has been proposed, to compare the effectiveness of different telestroke models, clinical management, and patient's outcomes.[15] To achieve this consensus, an international expert panel of clinicians, researchers, and managers from the Australasia Pacific region, US, United Kingdom, and Europe was convened. The final dataset included different variables including 12 categories: telestroke network/program details about initiating hospital, patient characteristics, presentation to hospital, general clinical care within the first 24 h, thrombolysis treatment, endovascular treatments, neurosurgery treatments, processes of care beyond 24 h, discharge information, postdischarge data, and follow-up data. As telemedicine intervention is likely to become more common in the future, coding for telemedicine including telestroke has been recently implemented with the International Classification of Health Interventions using the code XH01 for intervention or advice provided from a distant location, and the code XH02 for an intervention provided to a person or people in a distant location.[16] Remote neurological interventions, assessments, and advice provided by the remote physician to assist the emergency doctor in performing the thrombolysis can be quantified and analyzed for statistical purposes.

Other medical specialties

Telemedicine programs increase access to care in all clinical disciplines everywhere. Telemedicine is particularly suited to evaluating patients with Parkinson's disease (PD) and other movement disorders, primarily because much of the physical exam findings are visual. Telemedicine offers the opportunity for enhanced access to specialty care, thus potentially reducing the lack of diagnosis, delay in treatments, and subsequent morbidity and mortality, and improving quality of life for patients with PD and other movement disorders. In the US, the Department of Veterans Affairs (VA) Office of Connected Care leverages robust telemedicine infrastructure and advanced information technologies, including telehealth and mobile applications, to provide alternatives to in-person clinic visits.[17] These teleconsultations include not only synchronous encounters for patients at remote VA clinics, but home telehealth, and e-consultations as well. Kaiser Permanente, an integrated managed care consortium, has widely adopted a telehealth model accounting for more than half of all health encounters in the system in 2016.[18] Medicare, the United States' universal health care system for older (> 65 years of age) and disabled adults, currently reimburses telemedicine in only a subset of rural areas. Canada is also home to one of the most established telemedicine programs. This program offers telehealth visits from home as part of the armamentarium for caring for PD patients.[19] Deep brain stimulation (DBS) makers are also examining ways to remotely perform DBS programming for PD patients without requiring patients to leave their homes.[20] With regards to other movement disorders such as Huntington's disease (HD), in a survey conducted to analyze the organization of clinical services for HD at 231 sites surveyed in Europe, North America, Latin America, and Oceania, multidisciplinary case reviews were offered in 54.5% of sites, and only videoconferencing and telemedicine were used by only 23.6% of sites.[21]

Epilepsy remains an undertreated condition around the world, though efforts to improve epilepsy care have been promising in Western countries.[5] There are more than 50 million epilepsy patients in the world, with 85% living in developing countries, according to the WHO.[22] The WHO has suggested that nonphysician health workers should be empowered to diagnose and manage epilepsy; to do this, they will need considerable medical support, which might be provided by telemedicine through the telephone, smartphone applications, or a combination.[23] The application of store-and-forward technology for electroencephalography (EEG) interpretation is a reasonable alternative in some countries where neurophysiologists are not readily available. The feasibility of an EEG service between a community hospital and a tertiary hospital has been tested in Spain. Most of the patients (98%) were satisfied with the tele-EEG system in a 116-patient study, and 75% preferred it to the conventional consult, due to reduced traveling expenses and the total invested time in the EEG test.[5, 24]

Similarly, tele-EEG has been a timely and effective method of providing EEG services in the United Kingdom, especially for hospitals that cannot recruit neurophysiologists.[5, 25] In Canada, the feasibility of epilepsy care follow-up through teleneurology was tested in a study conducted by the University of Alberta hospital epilepsy clinic.[5, 26] About 90% of patients in both groups were satisfied with the quality of the service. A Canadian survey reported that a large number of neurologists (79.5%) had access to videoconferencing equipment.

Teleneurology toward a preventive medicine and interdisciplinary approach

Telemedicine has shown efficacy in the treatment of chronic diseases such as heart failure and high blood pressure.[27] Telemonitoring, for example, cardiovascular risk factors for stroke, or motor deterioration in PD, would facilitate early interventions and reduce the morbidity-mortality rate and the number of re-hospitalizations that directly correlate with social costs, and promoting a better quality of life. In Latin America, given the large and increasing burden of stroke, the GBD, Injuries, and Risk Factors 2017 study estimated that the prevention of attributable risk factors of stroke could reduce the stroke burden by 85.3% (95% uncertainty interval 82.6–87.8). The representative of ministries of 13 countries from Latin America participated in a meeting in Gramado, Brazil, in 2018 covering public stroke awareness, prevention strategies, delivery and organization of care, clinical practice gaps, and unmet needs. The meeting culminated with the adoption of the unique Gramado Declaration, signed by all ministerial officials who attended the meeting. The Gramado Declaration established priorities for stroke prevention and treatments to reduce the global and regional burden of stroke. In this declaration, the use of telemedicine was encouraged.[28, 29]

Several other projects have been developed in this field as well. In France, there are several telemedicine projects expanding and centered on the elderly designed to prevent mortality, morbidity, and the number of hospitalizations.[27] One of these projects is called "Telegeria," offering teleconsultations for elderly patients in geriatric hospitals and nursing homes based on the observation of polipathology and the occurrence of geriatric risks among the elderly, which requires multidisciplinary specialists including neurologists. As an example, a 15-month activity study identified 700 telemedicine sessions from retirement homes with hospital specialists involving different areas, ranging from orthopedics (35%) and cardiology (32%) to neurology (4%).[30]

One of the most successful and established models of regional care in PD is the ParkinsonNet model in the Netherlands,[19] where medical and allied health interventions are delivered within integrated regional community networks dispersed throughout the country by PD-specific therapists with specialized training who manage high caseloads.[31] Better quality of care, fewer PD-related complications, lower mortality risk, and lower total health care costs have been achieved compared to usual care. The use of specialized occupational therapy delivered in the community setting has resulted in an improvement in self-perceived daily functioning.[32] While ParkinsonNet has been introduced to other European countries such as Chzequia,[33] its applicability has limited generalization across other health care systems. Singapore has also been working toward an interdisciplinary approach for community care of PD patients that allows health care professionals to participate actively in the clinical care of these patients.[34]

Telemedicine programs in underserved areas

In low-income countries and other underserved areas, there are often large disparities in health care access between the rich and the poor, indicating that telemedicine could be open to most patients, regardless of wealth or status. Thus, in theory, telemedicine programs should represent an inexpensive and efficient way of extending medical care to remote and difficult-to-reach communities.[35] Unfortunately, in practice, telemedicine, including neurology programs, faces limitations, such as the high initial cost of setting up a scheme and the lack of local expertise required for the maintenance and repair of core equipment.[36] Key advantages of regional programs are the convenience for real-time teleconsultations (shared time zone and language) and the rapid patient referral to hub centers for further evaluation/ treatment.[36] There are several international programs designed to promote the use of teleneurology in underserved areas and developing countries. In this regard, a successful program developed in Albania and Cabo Verde was built by the Initiate-Build-Operate-Transfer (IBOT) strategy formulated by the International Virtual e-Hospital Foundation (IVeH) and with support from US government agencies such as the US Agency for International Development (USAID), Department of State, and United States European Command (EUCOM), and the Slovenian government (Ministry of Foreign Affairs), among other partners. Ratifi et al.[37] reviewed the similarities and differences between telemedicine programs in two different countries. Out of 2442 teleconsultations in Cabo Verde and 2724 teleconsultations in Albania between 2014 and 2018, radiology, neurotrauma, stroke, and general neurology, followed by cardiology and orthopedics, were the champion clinical disciplines in both countries.[37] This program, which was run progressively, reduced unnecessary and costly transfers, resulting in saved resources. According to the authors, the number of consultations reflects the lack of local specialty expertise to provide health care service, and it thus can be used as a model for establishing future planning and investment.[37]

In another review of teleconsultations performed by Gowda et al. for neurology services in rural and semiurban parts of India between 2010 and 2017, 189 teleneurology outpatient consultations were provided through the Tele-Medicine Centre, located at a tertiary hospital-based research center in southern India.[38] The most common diagnosis in these outpatient teleconsultations was a seizure disorder (17.5%), followed by cerebrovascular accident/stroke (14.8%). Interestingly, 87.3% were found to benefit from teleneurology consultations using interventions such as a change of medications (30.1%), referral to a specialist for review (15.8%), and further evaluation of illness and inpatient care (7.93%). Another study by Patterson et al., designed to compare referral patterns to the Swinfen Charitable Trust from the Middle East with those received from the rest of the developing world,[39] found that simple emails connecting doctors in the Middle East with specialists elsewhere in the world were feasible and sustainable over time, even in war-torn countries. For neurological cases, radiological images were attached to the referring email for 10 patients and eight patients' clinical images. The neurologist requested video clips for a further three patients. These consultations helped to diagnose brain tumors, demyelinating disease, conversion disorders, and, upon some other cases, referred to neuroradiology and neurosurgery opinions too.[39]

In terms of movement disorders, over the last 7 years, the International Parkinson's Disease and Movement Disorder Society has been sponsoring several teleneurology programs in underserved areas, including South America, Africa, and China. The Asynchronous Consultation in Movement Disorders (ACMD) is a specialized program conducted in Africa.

This store-and-forward technology has enabled referring sites with slower internet speeds and variable electrical power to participate in ACMD. In addition, the referring sites in Africa can access the simple equipment required (laptop, digital camera, or smartphone) to request a consultation, eliminating the challenges of scheduling virtual clinic visits in different time zones. The ACMD program is structured so that the consultant solely provides advice to the local provider, who continues to be the treating physician. The consultant's report may include differential diagnosis, a list of follow-up questions for consideration, and/or an empiric plan of care. The consultant can also attach other documents, such as relevant academic literature. The feedback from consultants and referrers has been overwhelmingly positive. In particular, the referrers have identified that the program has been especially useful as a professional development tool. In 2018, 12 out of 51 clinical cases (43%) presented using the ACMD platform were related to dystonia, myoclonus, and dyskinesias, and none contained queries regarding PD,[40] likely the most commonly discussed movement disorder elsewhere. These observations highlight the difficulties of diagnosing hyperkinetic movement disorders in underserved areas. A different project conducted in China was designed to provide care to PD patients through a network of neighborhood clinics and train primary care neurologists in neighborhood clinics to diagnose and manage PD with specialist support. The community neurologists were satisfied with the use of telemedicine to obtain expert advice. Although it was not statistically significant, a reduction in fractures, emergency visits, and hospitalizations was observed in the intervention group. The use of telemedicine facilitated consultations between community neurologists and movement disorders experts, providing a step forward in access to high-quality care in remote provinces of China.[35]

Humanitarian crisis

Humanitarian emergencies defined by armed conflict, political strife, famine, or natural disaster can devastate populations rapidly. Neurologic disorders accompany these complex humanitarian emergencies but often go unheeded, exacerbated by a scarcity of neurologists. Teleneurology offers the promise of neurologic care remotely in the face of this inadequate local clinician supply.[41] An international program conducted teleneurology consultations with Médecins Sans Frontières, a medical humanitarian emergency nonprofit organization with several projects in different countries across the world, in addition to their search and rescue operations.[42] In 2017, more than 150 consults were provided by > 10 neurologists with active medical license living in six countries, including three pediatric neurologists. Based on the Médecins Sans Frontières experience, the need for improved resource availability for neurologic disorders in resource-limited settings, and the importance of follow-up and feedback represent the potential areas of growth for future teleneurology projects in humanitarian crises.

On March 11, 2020, the WHO declared the coronavirus disease 2019 (COVID-19) outbreak as a pandemic. The response strategy included early diagnosis, patient isolation, symptomatic monitoring of contacts, suspected and confirmed cases, and public health quarantine.[43] The COVID-19 pandemic has resulted in millions of infections and hundreds of thousands of deaths worldwide,[44] despite community mitigation strategies to slow the transmission of disease and protect vulnerable populations.[45] As hospitals became overrun with COVID-19 patients, the risk of visits for care of other disorders began to outweigh the risk of deferred care or alternative approaches. In many centers, other inpatient admissions or surgeries have been limited to life-threatening conditions.

Telemedicine can also be used to address the ongoing health care needs of patients with chronic illnesses, including neurological disorders, to reduce in-person clinic visits. Such uses of telemedicine reduce human exposures (among health care workers and patients) to a range of infectious diseases and ensure that medical supplies are reserved for patients who need them.[46] Many European Union and Asian countries and the US have expanded laws and regulations to permit greater adoption of telemedicine systems, providing increased guidance on digital health technologies and cybersecurity expectations and expanded reimbursement options.[46] In this regard, many organizations, including the American Academy of Neurology and the International Parkinson and Movement Disorder Society, have issued telemedicine guidelines.[47, 48]

In an international survey developed by the Telemedicine Study Group of the International Parkinson's disease and movement disorder society,[49] four domains of telemedicine—legal regulations, reimbursement, clinical usage, and barriers—were compared prior to and during the COVID-19 pandemic. Data were obtained from 43 countries within Pan-America, Europe, Middle East, Africa, and Asia-Oceania. Overall, there was a vast global increase in all forms of telemedicine for movement disorders, across low-to-high income countries, as an immediate response to the COVID-19 pandemic. This increase in teleneurology uses was aided by the widespread availability of technology and changes in government regulations. However, issues of privacy concerns, variable internet connections, lack of reimbursement, and a desire for training in telemedicine visits were highlighted worldwide.

Questions remain about the longevity of changes in regulations and reimbursement practices as the world moves past the COVID-19 pandemic. The need for "social distancing" during the COVID-19 pandemic has created a significant surge in the number of teleneurology visits, which will probably continue for the next few months. It may have initiated a more permanent transition to virtual technology incorporated medical care.[50] Teleneurology, a solution for outpatient care during the COVID-19 pandemic, has been proposed for different neurological disorders. Different examples include: in Italy for dementia, amyotrophic lateral sclerosis, multiple sclerosis, frontotemporal lobar degeneration, and parkinsonism;[51–55] in the US and India, for general neurology including urgent and nonurgent visits[56–58]; in Asia for central nervous system inflammatory diseases[59]; in Spain for neuromuscular disorders and epilepsy[60, 61]; and in Saudi Arabia and Malaysia for stroke.[62, 63] In terms of neuropediatric disorders, a survey from different international epilepsy associations evaluated the effect of the COVID-19 pandemic on international access to care and practice patterns for children with epilepsy.[64] This study concluded that in response to COVID-19, pediatric epilepsy programs have implemented crisis standards of care that include increased telemedicine, decreased EEG use, changes in treatments of infantile spasms, and cessation of epilepsy surgery, causing profound changes to the care of children with epilepsy.

Education

Successful integration of teleneurology training into general practitioner and allied health professional programs is vital to expand access to neurologic care around the world as the societal demand for these services increases. International examples include the development of the outpatient teleneurology curriculum for residents in the US. Afshari et al. reported the utility, challenges, and benefits of teleneurology training in 11 neurology residents after 2–4 weeks of rotation. After completing this course, residents' performance on quizzes improved from 53% to 88% (p = 0.002), showing a statistically significant improvement in medical knowledge. The International Parkinson's Disease and Movement Disorder Society has sponsored several international tele-education programs in movement disorders. The first one, in 2014, using a teleneurology approach, including a tele-education PD program for health providers, was conducted at Hospital Laquintinie in Douala (Cameroon).[65] Twenty lectures over the course of a year connected participants with movement disorder experts using live, synchronous video conferences, and teaching materials. Thirty-three health professionals (52.4% women), including 16 doctors and 17 allied health professionals, and 18 speakers, participated. Videoconferences were successfully completed in 80%, participation ranged from 20% to 70%, and satisfaction was at least above average in 70% of participants. Whereas medical knowledge was dramatically improved, postcourse patient access was not changed in the short term.

The second project was conducted in 2016, using a different audience target: a movement disorders tele-education project for medical students was conducted in a low-middle-income country (Cameroon) and a middle-high-income country (Argentina) lacking access to movement disorders education.[66] Six real-time videoconferences covering hyperkinetic and hypokinetic movement disorders were included. This study included 151 undergraduate medical students (79.4% from Argentina, 20.6% from Cameroon). Feasibility was acceptable with 100% and 85.7% of the videoconferences completed in Argentina and Cameroon, respectively, and medical knowledge improved similarly in both countries. Attendance was higher in Argentina compared to Cameroon (75% vs. 33.1%). The third program was started in 2018, and the results have not been published yet. In this program, called the Center to Center Movement Disorders Training Program, one academic center will partner up to two centers in underserved regions to develop movement disorders expertise in an underserved region.

Conclusion

Setting up any telemedicine program requires complex, multilevel partnerships between organizations from different sectors. Collaborating with the government allows the program to reach a massive scale and secure subsidies in costs to keep the end-user price low and provide health care at reduced rates for the poorest. Teleneurology is expanding across the world, facilitating the access of low-income countries and other underserved areas to neurological services. Several telemedicine studies for clinical care and education have been conducted, showing feasibility and high satisfaction in different neurology specialties and during a humanitarian crisis. With advances in the development of mobile communications in the future, there is no doubt that teleneurology will have a more significant impact on the delivery of health care around the world.

References

1. https://www.Who.Int/goe/publications/goe_telemedicine_2010.pdf (Accessed 24 July 2020).
2. Janca A, Aarli JA, Prilipko L, Dua T, Saxena S, Saraceno B. Who/wfn survey of neurological services: a worldwide perspective. *J Neurol Sci.* 2006;247:29–34.
3. Group GBDNDC. Global, regional, and national burden of neurological disorders during 1990-2015: a systematic analysis for the global burden of disease study 2015. *Lancet Neurol.* 2017;16:877–897.
4. Collaborators GBDN. Global, regional, and national burden of neurological disorders, 1990-2016: a systematic analysis for the global burden of disease study 2016. *Lancet Neurol.* 2019;18:459–480.
5. Khalid S, Varade P, Bhattacharya P, Madhavan R. International teleneurology. In: Tsao J, Demaerschalk B, eds. *Teleneurology in Practice.* New York, NY: Springer; 2015. https://doi.org/10.1007/978-1-4939-2349-6_2.
6. Wardlaw JM, Murray V, Berge E, et al. Recombinant tissue plasminogen activator for acute ischaemic stroke: an updated systematic review and meta-analysis. *Lancet.* 2012;379:2364–2372.
7. Levine SR, Gorman M. "Telestroke": the application of telemedicine for stroke. *Stroke.* 1999;30:464–469.
8. Schwamm LH, Holloway RG, Amarenco P, et al. A review of the evidence for the use of telemedicine within stroke systems of care: a scientific statement from the American Heart Association/American Stroke Association. *Stroke.* 2009;40:2616–2634.
9. Kepplinger J, Barlinn K, Deckert S, Scheibe M, Bodechtel U, Schmitt J. Safety and efficacy of thrombolysis in telestroke: a systematic review and meta-analysis. *Neurology.* 2016;87:1344–1351.
10. *Hawke's Bay's Teleradiology Service is Safe.* Available from: http://www.Scoop.Co.Nz/stories/ge0609/s00009/hawkes-bays-teleradiology-service-is-safe.Htm. Accessed 12 August 2020.
11. Ranta A, Lanford J, Busch S, et al. Impact and implementation of a sustainable regional telestroke network. *Intern Med J.* 2017;47:1270–1275.
12. Vatankhah B, Schenkel J, Furst A, Haberl RL, Audebert HJ. Telemedically provided stroke expertise beyond normal working hours. The telemedical project for integrative stroke care. *Cerebrovasc Dis.* 2008;25:332–337.
13. Ranta A, Busch S. Impact of discontinuation of telestroke: the nelson experience. *N Z Med J.* 2018;131:29–34.
14. Bladin CF, Moloczij N, Ermel S, et al. Victorian stroke telemedicine project: implementation of a new model of translational stroke care for Australia. *Intern Med J.* 2015;45:951–956.
15. Cadilhac DA, Bagot KL, Demaerschalk BM, et al. Establishment of an internationally agreed minimum data set for acute telestroke. *J Telemed Telecare.* 2020;,1357633X19899262.
16. Ohannessian R, Fortune N, Moulin T, Madden R. Telemedicine, telestroke, and artificial intelligence can be coded with the international classification of health interventions. *Telemed J E Health.* 2020;26:574–575.
17. U.S. Department of Veterans Affairs. *Fy 2018/fy 2016: annual performance plan and report.* Available from: Https://www.Va.Gov/budget/docs/vaapprfy2018.Pdf. Accessed 15 November 2017.

18. Https://mhealthintelligence.Com/news/kaiser-ceo-telehealth-outpaced-in-person-visits-last-year (Accessed 10 January 2018).
19. Bloem BR, Munneke M. Revolutionising management of chronic disease: the parkinsonnet approach. *BMJ.* 2014;348:g1838.
20. Li D, Zhang C, Gault J, et al. Remotely programmed deep brain stimulation of the bilateral subthalamic nucleus for the treatment of primary Parkinson disease: a randomized controlled trial investigating the safety and efficacy of a novel deep brain stimulation system. *Stereotact Funct Neurosurg.* 2017;95:174–182.
21. Frich JC, Rae D, Roxburgh R, et al. Health care delivery practices in Huntington's disease specialty clinics: an international survey. *J Huntingtons Dis.* 2016;5:207–213.
22. Decapua J. *Epilepsy Burdens Developing Countries.* http://www.Voanews.Com/content/epilepsy-deve-world-2oct12/1518932.html. Accessed 23 July 2020.
23. Patterson V. Managing epilepsy by telemedicine in resource-poor settings. *Front Public Health.* 2019;7:321.
24. Lasierra N, Alesanco A, Campos C, Caudevilla E, Fernandez J, Garcia J. Experience of a real-time tele-eeg service. *Conf Proc IEEE Eng Med Biol Soc.* 2009;2009:5211–5214.
25. Coates S, Clarke A, Davison G, Patterson V. Tele-eeg in the UK: a report of over 1,000 patients. *J Telemed Telecare.* 2012;18:243–246.
26. Ahmed SN, Mann C, Sinclair DB, et al. Feasibility of epilepsy follow-up care through telemedicine: a pilot study on the patient's perspective. *Epilepsia.* 2008;49:573–585.
27. Zulfiqar AA, Hajjam A, Andres E. Focus on the different projects of telemedicine centered on the elderly in France. *Curr Aging Sci.* 2019;11:202–215.
28. Collaborators GBDS. Global, regional, and national burden of stroke, 1990–2016: a systematic analysis for the global burden of disease study 2016. *Lancet Neurol.* 2019;18:439–458.
29. Ouriques Martins SC, Sacks C, Hacke W, et al. Priorities to reduce the burden of stroke in Latin American countries. *Lancet Neurol.* 2019;18:674–683.
30. Espinoza P, Gouaze A, Bonnet B, et al. Deployment of telemedicine in health territory. Tele-geria, a precursor experimental model. *Telemed Health.* 2011;725:9–17.
31. Nijkrake MJ, Keus SH, Overeem S, et al. The Parkinsonnet concept: development, implementation and initial experience. *Mov Disord.* 2010;25:823–829.
32. Ypinga JHL, de Vries NM, Boonen L, et al. Effectiveness and costs of specialised physiotherapy given via Parkinsonnet: a retrospective analysis of medical claims data. *Lancet Neurol.* 2018;17:153–161.
33. Gal O, Srp M, Konvalinkova R, et al. Physiotherapy in Parkinson's disease: building Parkinsonnet in Czechia. *Parkinsons Dis.* 2017;2017:8921932.
34. Aye YM, Liew S, Neo SX, et al. Patient-centric care for Parkinson's disease: from hospital to the community. *Front Neurol.* 2020;11:502.
35. Ben-Pazi H, Browne P, Chan P, et al. The promise of telemedicine for movement disorders: an interdisciplinary approach. *Curr Neurol Neurosci Rep.* 2018;18:26.
36. Khanal S, Burgon J, Leonard S, Griffiths M, Eddowes LA. Recommendations for the improved effectiveness and reporting of telemedicine programs in developing countries: results of a systematic literature review. *Telemed J E Health.* 2015;21:903–915.
37. Latifi R, Azevedo V, Boci A, Parsikia A, Latifi F, Merrell RC. Telemedicine consultation as an indicator of local telemedicine champions' contributions, health care system needs or both: Tales from two continents. *Telemed J E Health.* 2020.
38. Gowda GS, Manjunatha N, Kulkarni K, et al. A collaborative tele-neurology outpatient consulation service in Karnataka: seven years of experience from a tele-medicine center. *Neurol India.* 2020;68:358–363.
39. Patterson V, Swinfen P, Swinfen R, Azzo E, Taha H, Wootton R. Supporting hospital doctors in the middle east by email telemedicine: something the industrialized world can do to help. *J Med Internet Res.* 2007;9, e30.

40. Srinivasan R, Ben-Pazi H, Dekker M, et al. Telemedicine for hyperkinetic movement disorders. *Tremor Other Hyperkinet Mov (NY)*. 2020;10. https://doi.org/10.7916/tohm. v0.698.

41. Saadi A, Mateen FJ. International issues: teleneurology in humanitarian crises: lessons from the medecins sans frontieres experience. *Neurology*. 2017;89:e16–e19.

42. Medicine Sans frontieres. www.msf.org. Accessed 8 August 2020.

43. Ohannessian R, Duong TA, Odone A. Global telemedicine implementation and integration within health systems to fight the covid-19 pandemic: a call to action. *JMIR Public Health Surveill*. 2020;6, e18810.

44. World Health Organization. *Coronavirus disease 2019 (covid-19) situation report—97*; 2020. https://www.Who.Int/docs/default-source/corona wirrell et al 9viruse/situation-reports/20200426-sitrep-97-covid-19.pdf. Accessed 30 July 2020.

45. Centers for Disease Control and Prevention. *Community Mitigation*; 2020. https://www. Cdc.Gov/coronavirus/2019-ncov/php/openamerica/community-mitigation.Html. Accessed 30 July 2020.

46. Rockwell KL, Gilroy AS. Incorporating telemedicine as part of covid-19 outbreak response systems. *Am J Manag Care*. 2020;26:147–148.

47. Telemedicine in Your Movement Disorders Practice. Available from: https://www. movementdisorders.org/mds/about/committees–other-groups/telemedicine-in-your-movement-disorders-practice-a-step-by-step-guide.htm (Accessed 22 July 2020).

48. *Telemedicine and Covid-19 Implementation Guide*. Available from: https://www.aan.com/ siteassets/home-page/tools-and-resources/practicing-neurologist- -administrators/tele-medicine-and-remote-care/20-telemedicine-and-covid19-v103.pdf. Accessed 22 July 2020.

49. Hassan A, Mari Z, Gatto E, et al. Global survey on telemedicine utilization for movement disorders during the covid-19 pandemic. *Mov Disord*. 2020;35:1701-1711.

50. Roy B, Nowak RJ, Roda R, et al. Teleneurology during the covid-19 pandemic: a step forward in modernizing medical care. *J Neurol Sci*. 2020;414:116930.

51. Cuffaro L, Di Lorenzo F, Bonavita S, Tedeschi G, Leocani L, Lavorgna L. Dementia care and covid-19 pandemic: a necessary digital revolution. *Neurol Sci*. 2020;41:1977–1979.

52. Capozzo R, Zoccolella S, Musio M, Barone R, Accogli M, Logroscino G. Telemedicine is a useful tool to deliver care to patients with amyotrophic lateral sclerosis during covid-19 pandemic: results from southern Italy. *Amyotroph Lateral Scler Frontotemporal Degener*. 2020;21:542–548.

53. Moccia M, Lanzillo R, Brescia Morra V, et al. Assessing disability and relapses in multiple sclerosis on tele-neurology. *Neurol Sci*. 2020;41:1369–1371.

54. Capozzo R, Zoccolella S, Frisullo ME, et al. Telemedicine for delivery of care in frontotemporal lobar degeneration during covid-19 pandemic: results from southern Italy. *J Alzheimers Dis*. 2020;76:481–489.

55. Cilia R, Mancini F, Bloem BR, Eleopra R. Telemedicine for parkinsonism: a two-step model based on the covid-19 experience in Milan, Italy. *Parkinsonism Relat Disord*. 2020;75:130–132.

56. Grossman SN, Han SC, Balcer LJ, et al. Rapid implementation of virtual neurology in response to the covid-19 pandemic. *Neurology*. 2020;94:1077–1087.

57. Punia V, Nasr G, Zagorski V, et al. Evidence of a rapid shift in outpatient practice during the covid-19 pandemic using telemedicine. *Telemed J E Health*. 2020.

58. Ganapathy K. Telemedicine and neurological practice in the covid-19 era. *Neurol India*. 2020;68:555–559.

59. Viswanathan S. Management of idiopathic cns inflammatory diseases during the covid-19 pandemic: perspectives and strategies for continuity of care from a south east asian center with limited resources. *Mult Scler Relat Disord*. 2020;44:102353.

60. Romero-Imbroda J, Reyes-Garrido V, Ciano-Petersen NL, Serrano-Castro PJ. Emergency implantation of a teleneurology service at the neuromuscular unit of hospital regional de malaga during the sars-cov-2 pandemic. *Neurologia*. 2020;35:415–417.

61. Hernando-Requejo V, Huertas-Gonzalez N, Lapena-Motilva J, Ogando-Duran G. The epilepsy unit during the covid-19 epidemic: the role of telemedicine and the effects of confinement on patients with epilepsy. *Neurologia*. 2020;35:274–276.

62. Alzahrani SS, Aleisa FK, Alghalbi JA, et al. Stroke management pathway during covid-19 pandemic scientific statement by the saudi stroke society. *Neurosciences (Riyadh)*. 2020;25:226–229.

63. Wan Asyraf WZ, Ah Khan YK, Chung LW, et al. Malaysia stroke council guide on acute stroke care service during covid-19 pandemic. *Med J Malaysia*. 2020;75:311–313.

64. Wirrell EC, Grinspan ZM, Knupp KG, et al. Care delivery for children with epilepsy during the covid-19 pandemic: an international survey of clinicians. *J Child Neurol*. 2020;, 883073820940189.

65. Cubo E, Doumbe J, Njiengwe E, et al. A Parkinson's disease tele-education program for health care providers in Cameroon. *J Neurol Sci*. 2015;357:285–287.

66. Cubo E, Doumbe J, Lopez E, et al. Telemedicine enables broader access to movement disorders curricula for medical students. *Tremor Other Hyperkinet Mov (NY)*. 2017;7:501.

CHAPTER 18

Future of telemedicine

Robert L. Satcher, Jr, MD, PhD
MD Anderson Cancer Center, Houston, TX, United States

Telemedicine (also known as telehealth, as will be used interchangeably in this chapter) is the remote provision of health care using any variety of telecommunication tools, wearable devices, computing technology, and/ or robotic technology. Telecommunication tools can include smartphones, mobile devices, tablets, and telephones, with or without a video connection. Telemedicine usage has grown rapidly in response to the COVID-19 pandemic, as social distancing and quarantine have limited access to routine medical care. The subsequent expansion in telemedicine use has ushered in a long-anticipated technology-driven era of health care. In the near future, the use of telehealth is expected to expand the reach of medical care, by routinely reaching those with access to telecommunications technologies. Although there have been publications that have examined the current and historical use of telemedicine, few have focused on its evolution and future.[1–3] Here, we examine the factors that are shaping the practice, limitations, and future adoption of telemedicine.

Background/past implementation

The earliest applications of telemedicine were for providing care to the military, prisoners, and patients in rural locations.[3] Telemedicine was also (and continues to be) famously used to provide care to astronauts during spaceflight.[4,5] Accordingly, its applications remained restricted to these groups rather than gaining further traction more widely. Reimbursement was limited to patient care scenarios defined by remote location, thereby constraining the widespread use of telehealth. Legal issues also contributed to limited implementation, with state licensure laws restricting health care professionals to practicing in the state in which a patient is located when medical services are rendered. An overview of the limitations of telemedicine, and how they have evolved, is shown in Table 18.1. Prior to the pandemic, more than any other factors, reimbursement and legal constraints dominated the telemedicine landscape, constraining further expansion.[6,7]

Table 18.1 Factors limiting telemedicine adoption, with predicted future evolution.

	Limitations and predicted evolution		
	Early/Past	Present/Current	Future
Reimbursement	Fragmented insurance coverage	Pandemic driven	Continued Medicare and Medicaid coverage policy, level uncertain
Clinical quality	Quality of patient–physician relationship thought to be less c/w in-person visit	Empirical equivalence; surveys show comfort with video visits by both patients and physicians	Further technological enhancement of virtual visits using AI, robotics, and tele-communications that are more intuitive and convenient
	Potential for overprescribing and similar abuse	Optimize care model	Mixture of in-patient and virtual visits that minimize risk
Legal issues	State-by-state licensing requirement	Pandemic relaxation of licensing requirement	Implement interstate medical licensure compact and/or TELE-MED Act of 2015, federal legislation that provides national licensing for telemedicine practice
Social issues	Limited access to internet/mobile phones	Increasing broadband access	High access nationally, including underserved communities

Patient care quality concerns have also been a focus. The virtual nature of telemedicine has the potential to compromise the quality of patient-physician interaction, and reduce the quality of care.[3] Concerns about performing remote patient assessments, especially with patients where there was no prior established relationship, contributed to hesitancy in expanding the use of telemedicine. It was hypothesized that these encounters could lead to inappropriate care (i.e., excessive use of antibiotics), create shallow patient-physician relationships, increase liability from overprescription, etc., and detract from integrated and coordinated care.[3]

The groundwork for the expansion of telehealth lay in the advancement of communication technology and the internet. The conversion to electronic health records and the development of mobile phones and smartphones created the platform required for video visits, removing the principle technological constraint to widespread usage, and importantly, promoting a comfort level with using video as a substitute for in person interaction. Some of the earliest successful applications included the use of telehealth for acute conditions, such as trauma and stroke.[8] The telestroke program, which provided acute stroke care from a remote neurologist to a patient in an emergency department, became mainstream following its introduction in 1999.[8] The largest care provider for patients with stroke in the US is currently a telemedicine company rather than a major medical center.[9] Other areas of past usage were mental health, school visits by medical assistants, video calls, telephone calls, care for episodic conditions such as sinusitis, and asynchronous monitoring of chronic conditions.[10–13] Despite these successes, a plateau had been reached in the use of telemedicine. Other benefits of wider usage, such as cost reduction, increased access to care, and convenience, remained theoretical, with no data to substantiate predictions. The big change occurred with the COVID-19 pandemic.[6,7]

Current environment

The COVID-19 crisis catalyzed the use of telemedicine, with adoption by major hospital centers, and expansion to application in complex care models such as cancer care and neurologic disorders.[6] The first big adjustment that created this change was with reimbursement. Insurance coverage was previously fragmented, with 29 states having telehealth parity laws requiring that private insurers cover telehealth services to the same extent as in-person care.[14] With Medicaid, 48 states covered telehealth services. However, Medicare only reimbursed clinical facilities in areas that had a shortage of health care providers.[15] As of 2012, Medicare only spent \$5 M (0.001% of total expenditure) on telemedicine services.[15] However, in 2020, telehealth coverage was expanded in response to the pandemic. Under the Coronavirus Preparedness and Response Supplemental Appropriations Act 2020, the Centers for Medicare and Medicaid Services (CMS) waived key telehealth requirements, allowing Medicare beneficiaries to receive services from their homes with fewer restrictions.[16] The US requirement that the patient and clinician must be in the same state was lifted for both Medicare and Medicaid, but not for those with private or no insurance.[6,16] Medicare thus began reimbursing telehealth services for the same dollar amount as in-person visits. In response, private insurers also began to reimburse telehealth.

The second big adjustment was to state licensure requirements. Current guidelines require providers to have licenses in each state in which they practice, a costly and time-consuming issue for health systems that span several states and telehealth services that reach patients regardless of where they are located. There has yet to be agreement about how best to manage the issue, with some supporting the current practice, some supporting licensure compacts that span several states or regions, and some even suggesting one license for the entire country.

In response, some states relaxed their guidelines during the ongoing COVID-19 crisis, but providers noted that the process was confusing and nonuniform, with each state having its own rules, such as the necessity of obtaining temporary licenses to practice telemedicine in some states.[17,18] Moreover, those emergency measures were slated to end with the emergency.

Prior to the pandemic, the Department of Veterans Affairs was the only exception to licensing restrictions. The Veterans E-Health and Telemedicine Support (VETS) Act in 2017 granted VAMC physicians approval to treat veterans in any location via telehealth. Recently, there were two bills introduced to Congress that would enable all providers to use telehealth in any state during the coronavirus pandemic. Both the Temporary Reciprocity to Ensure Access to Treatment (TREAT) Act and the Equal Access to Care Act are pending approval (as of this publication) and waive licensing restrictions temporarily.[19]

Nonetheless, the overall response triggered by Medicare reimbursement for telemedicine was the widespread, rapid adoption of telemedicine by most major health care centers as part of the clinical practice, not just in rural areas.[6,19] Predating the pandemic, Kaiser Permanente of Northern California was the largest organization, outside of the Department of Defense and the Department of Veterans Affairs, to cover the use of telehealth to improve care quality and reduce costs.[11] It provoked extensive adoption of telehealth visits within Kaiser, and empirical confirmation of its value, as measured by quality metrics and cost reductions.[20] In 2016, Kaiser had more virtual visits than in-person visits.[20]

Subsequent to pandemic provisions, many large organizations have become adopters of telehealth. Notably, the country's largest cancer hospital, the UT MD Anderson Cancer Center (MDACC), went from little to no activity to providing 25%–30% of ambulatory care using video visits, as of the time of this publication.[21] Another prescient example is with chronic neurological disorders. Individuals with neurological diseases are at increased risk when coinfected with COVID-19 because of their advanced age (e.g., Alzheimer's), comorbid conditions (e.g., respiratory impairment in amyotrophic lateral sclerosis), or immunosuppressive treatments.[6] To mitigate risk, telemedicine and remote home monitoring have been used to continue care. As a result, awareness has grown that this model has advantages that will continue post-pandemic, such as: (1) telemedicine facilitates care that is delivered close to the patient's home, reducing the risk for events such as falls or seizures; (2) treatment responses that are challenging to capture during episodic outpatient visits are more likely to be observed at home due to more frequent monitoring; (3) home monitoring also permits better observations of treatment outcomes, as with Parkinson's disease patients, who episodically can move well when observed by clinicians; (4) home environments provide greater confidentiality (useful because clinic visits can be associated with stigma); and (5) reducing inefficient and at times unsafe outpatient clinic visits, which can require individuals to travel long distances and incur considerable expense[6]. Consequently, telehealth startups are increasingly targeting large self-insured employers, health care organizations, and hospital systems with services ranging from video visits to remote monitoring and patient education.[20] This large-scale movement into telehealth has suddenly brought new focus to evaluation of mostly unproven care models for increasing access and improving patient health.

The initial returns on the telemedicine experience for providers and patients have been encouraging. In unpublished surveys of patient experiences, many patients now have an enhanced understanding of the need for remote visits.[21] There are empirical reports of care delivered remotely that reinforce its effectiveness, such as in the delivery of bad news.[1,2,6,7,22] Many patients surveyed prefer to receive bad news in the safety of their homes, rather than in the more impersonal clinic environment.[2] Moreover, many components of the physical exam, such as simple neurological assessments or examination of wounds following surgery, can be performed remotely.[3,23]

Another past concern was that telemedicine could only be used with patients who are tech-savvy. This has also had less impact than anticipated. Older and less tech-savvy patients have proven to be more adaptable than expected.[7] Moreover, reimbursement was added to include telephone calls for telemedicine care to ameliorate the issue of proficiency with mobile devices.[19] In general, many older adults are now accustomed to using smartphones or videoconferencing.[24]

Overall, the rapid expansion of telehealth into current daily medical practices across all specialties comes with challenges that will shape future adoption (Table 18.1). The prediction that technology will transform health care is finally becoming reality. Evidence abounds that we are experiencing a "tipping point" in telehealth, in which adoption moves beyond early adopters to the majority.[25] This rapid adoption is an indication of overdue investment in improving the delivery of health care. Over the last few decades, the health care industry lagged behind in investing in technology and innovation, ranking 19th among 22 major industries.[26] This translated into less than 30 cents out of every $100 spent on health care.[26] Not surprisingly, because of the unrealized potential for innovation, venture capital funding in digital health and technology has accelerated, reaching $9.5 billion in 2018, compared with $4.3 billion in 2015 (with a total of $58 billion invested in digital health companies since 2010).[27] Among the top funded categories, telemedicine was first, followed by data analytics, mHealth apps, clinical decision support, and mobile wireless technology.[28]

The current period is thus perhaps most accurately characterized as the inception of telehealth in the US medical system. Indeed, the future is likely to bring increased investment and technological advances, with opportunities for quality improvement and cost savings.

Future development and adoption

With an increasingly older population, the prevalence of illnesses such as Alzheimer's, cancer, cerebrovascular accidents, diabetes, chronic renal failure, and cardiac illnesses, will create new challenges for delivering quality care and containing costs. Predictions for the future of telemedicine are driven by the desire to identify innovative solutions that center on prevention, personalized diagnosis and treatment, and sustainable costs.[1] Overall, it is widely accepted that telemedicine will continue as part of medical practice at higher levels than prior to the pandemic. Telemedicine for common conditions, chronic conditions, and complex disorders should become part of the new normal rather than the exception.[1,3,6] The trends that will likely be the most influential for the future of telemedicine are linked, and have been the subject of previous reviews.[7,24] A summary of these and emerging new trends is shown in Table 18.2.

Table 18.2 Trends shaping telemedicine.

Trends	
Past/Present/Ongoing[3]	Future
Transformation from increasing access to convenience and cost reduction	Transformation to technology-driven innovation in health care (telecommunications devices, robotics)
Addressing chronic conditions using telemedicine care models	Multidisciplinary coordinated care with all specialties
Migration of telemedicine from hospitals to home applications	Personalized medicine (AI, cognitive computing)

In an article that focused on the state of telehealth from 2016, Dorsey et al. concluded that telehealth would expand as the digital divide decreased, and as smartphones became more ubiquitous.[3] In discussing relevant trends shaping telemedicine, the most important centered around the shift from increasing access to health care to providing convenience and reducing costs.[7] That trend has been accelerated in the current environment, and will continue to affect telemedicine for the foreseeable future. It is clear that telemedicine increases access, a point brought into focus by the pandemic. In addition, it is anticipated that costs will be lower, although the data to verify this prediction are only now becoming available. Numerous organizations, from academic health centers to private hospitals, now offer low-cost virtual visits.[11,29] Moreover, these visits are more convenient that in-person appointments for patients. Traditional visits, once scheduled, take an average of 20 days to be seen, with travel and wait times that routinely consume 2 h.[29] In contrast, telemedicine visits routinely occur around the clock at the request of the patient.[11] Because of this obvious advantage, interest has continued to grow in whether telemedicine practice models help to reduce health care costs. Empirically this seems to be the case, and in the future more telemedicine delivery models will incorporate the lessons derived from current applications.

Another important present and future trend is in using telemedicine for chronic conditions in addition to acute conditions, such as trauma and stroke.[8] Telehealth use for chronic conditions has increased substantially during the pandemic. The impetus predates recent events, as chronic conditions are estimated to affect more than 140 million people in the US, and account for 80% of health care expenditure.[30] The evidence to support the effectiveness and feasibility of telemedicine care for chronic conditions has grown steadily. As an example, a recent study showed that remote care by a neurologist using videoconferencing yielded outcomes comparable to regular outpatient visits, with much greater efficiency as measured by cost and time.[31] Other studies have demonstrated the utility of using telemedicine to deliver care in the home[32] and via remote monitoring.[33] Both passive and active monitoring are effective, as are real-time and store-forward formats. A recent report showed the effectiveness of e-diaries, which remotely screen for development or progression of nonmotor symptoms, such as pain, constipation, migraines, and seizures.[34,35] In other subspecialties (such as orthopedics) remote monitoring can be used to monitor recovery of mobility and function after surgery,[36,37] and for cancer patients, home monitoring is being actively evaluated for patients undergoing treatment such as chemotherapy, to reduce the risk of hospitalization by more precise and frequent intervention to mitigate side effects.[38] As cited by others, this persuasive evidence has not yet led to widespread adoption in everyday medical care, due to the cultural issue of resistance to change in the medical field.[6] However, these barriers are steadily falling, and in the future, since most experience to date has been positive, we expect to see continued expansion and adoption in all specialties.[3,6,36,38]

An additional trend that is accelerating is the migration of care away from hospitals and clinics to home. Underlying this trend is that historically, the gold standard for care was the house call, in which physicians came to see patients in their homes.[11] In the 1930s, 40% of physician-patient encounters occurred in the home.[39] A study of the prevalence of house calls in 1993 showed that, as a practice, the number of house calls by physicians has declined dramatically during the last 100 years.[39] Currently, a very small percentage (36,000 visits to 12,000 of 1.4 million patients, or 0.88%) of elderly Medicare patients (mainly those who are near the end of life) receive house calls from physicians.[11,39] Thus, telemedicine, interestingly, provides a benefit in delivering care that is closer to the house call model than other current hospital and clinic based models. Telemedicine essentially allows physicians to reenter the home. The interactions between patients and physicians is rebalanced and more equal as both parties are seated at eye level, and both parties are in environments that are comfortable[3], and since the most important aspect of making a diagnosis is history taking, the video visit model is as effective from this perspective as an in-person visit.[40,41] Data from numerous studies have begun to confirm that although the nature of the patient visit will change because of telehealth, by leveraging the unique strengths to define new care models, overall outcomes can be improved. For example, more frequent, shorter visits, can be accomplished, and combined with data collected more frequently and comprehensively using wearable monitors.[6,36]

The future will be affected by additional trends that are now coming into focus (Table 18.2). Telemedicine has long offered convenience, comfort, and confidentiality, with the promise of improving quality while reducing costs.[7,23] In light of the instantaneous transformation ushered in by the pandemic, telemedicine is no longer a niche practice, but minimally is beginning to compete with traditional in-person means of providing care. Thus, technology innovation can henceforth be expected to be central to the transformation of health care. Smartphones, which are increasingly available, can and will be used to expand access to underserved communities.[7] It is estimated that over 77% of Americans have smartphones. Smartphone ownership worldwide at the end of 2020 was 45% of the population.[42] As technology advances, there will be an increasingly sophisticated set of tools that harness the access provided by mobile smartphones, enable monitoring a person's health passively, and facilitate diagnosis and care interventions.

One can also envision the increased use of actuating technologies, such as robotics, in delivering health care in more convenient, home-based scenarios. As robots become more humanoid, a logical endpoint is a robotic/android personal health care assistant that not only monitors an individual's health, but also intervenes as required to arrange appointments, obtain prescriptions, and coordinate recommendations for dietary and lifestyle interventions. These enhanced capabilities will also bring heightened privacy concerns and unintended consequences, such as overreliance on technology for monitoring health, and profit driven use of unproven technology (similar to pharmaceuticals), necessitating additional regulations.[3,11,38]

An additional developing trend impacting the future is the desire to provide coordinated care. There are numerous specialties, such as cancer care, that are best practiced with a coordinated multidisciplinary strategy. For example, a patient who is being seen for lung cancer, may need to receive care from numerous physicians, including medical oncologists, radiation oncologists, and oncology surgeons.[38] On the diagnostic side, pathologists and radiologists may be involved, with a critical need for interaction with the care team to identify the best medical strategy. The patient's care program may also involve palliative care physicians, rehabilitation physicians, physical and occupational therapists, pharmacologists, and mental health care. For in-person visits (the current model of care), care coordination can be challenging, requiring multiple appointments and carefully executed team communication to ensure that plans are implemented as intended. Replicating this model with telemedicine will therefore be challenging. However, there are multiple possibilities for proceeding, ranging from having multidisciplinary virtual visits, where multiple specialists simultaneously visit with a patient and coordinate care, to combining remote visits with in-person visits to maximize efficiency. Technological innovation, specifically with artificial intelligence (AI), will facilitate the development of these approaches, and help to identify the optimal mixture of virtual and in-person appointments.[43]

AI is defined as an area of study engaging computers in human processes, such as learning, reasoning, or storing knowledge.[44] In the near future, AI techniques, such as machine learning, deep learning, and cognitive computing, may play a critical role in the evolution of telemedicine. There have been numerous proposed pathways for incorporating AI to optimize clinical management of chronic and complex diseases.[44] As proposed, AI uses sophisticated algorithms to analyze large volumes of patient data, thereby optimizing decision-making and clinical outcomes.[1,43,44] Some machine learning (ML) techniques (another AI subdiscipline) are being developed to automate decision support systems and facilitate diagnosis and/or prognosis estimation.[44] To date, AI has been used primarily for precision cardiovascular medicine,[43] but has the potential to exploit the potential of big data such as "omics" data, microbiome sequencing, and data collected from wearable devices and social media, which have previously been too large and complex to be used in real time.[43] Overall, these AI and ML strategies are in the early stages of development, and much more work is needed to define which patients will benefit from telemedicine solutions based on this technology.[1,44]

Lastly, an increasingly important trend affecting the future of telemedicine/telehealth is the emergence of predictive, personalized, preventive, and participatory (P4) medicine.[1] The P4 approach integrates complex biological data, as well as individual genome sequences, to better define health and well-being of an individual, with the purpose of predicting illness and for directing medical interventions.[45,46] As indicated in a recent review by Alonso et al., "P4 medicine currently promises to provide a revolutionary new biomedical focus that is holistic instead of reductionist".[1] Telemedicine and eHealth are essential for achieving this evolutionary step. The future of health care centers on offering patients a complete image of factors affecting their health, including real time analysis of biological information that is primarily gathered via telemedicine applications.[1,36,38,44] These biological data include genome, transcriptomic, proteomic, metabonomic, and interactomic information. Real-time and integrated analysis of this omics data is the best way of describing and treating patients, understanding illness, and specifically identifying personalized and applicable health treatments and prevention strategies.

Overall, the convergence of increasing demand for convenient health care, the ubiquity of technological tools that provide the ability to connect patients with care providers, and the accelerating presence of technology in health care points to a future in which telemedicine/telehealth will play a larger role. Governments, health care systems, and payers should be encouraged to institute the necessary policy, regulations, and practice models that embrace the new age of access from home and "medical care anywhere," that continues after the pandemic concludes.

References

1. Alonso SG, de la Torre Díez I, Zapiraín BG. Predictive, personalized, preventive and participatory (4P) medicine applied to telemedicine and eHealth in the literature. *J Med Syst.* 2019;43:140.
2. Barello S, et al. eHealth for patient engagement: a systematic review. *Front Psychol.* 2015;6:2013.
3. Dorsey ER, Topol EJ. State of telehealth. *N Engl J Med.* 2016;375:154–161.
4. Godard B. Innovation in healthcare in space to improve life on earth. *Soins.* 2019;64:18–23.
5. Grigoriev AI, Orlov OI. Telemedicine and spaceflight. *Aviat Space Environ Med.* 2002;73:688–693.
6. Bloem BR, Dorsey ER, Okun MS. The coronavirus disease 2019 crisis as catalyst for telemedicine for chronic neurological disorders. *JAMA Neurol.* 2020;77:927–928.
7. Dorsey ER, Okun MS, Bloem BR. Care, convenience, comfort, confidentiality, and contagion: the 5 C's that will shape the future of telemedicine. *J Parkinsons Dis.* 2020;10:893–897.
8. Levine SR, Gorman M. "Telestroke": the application of telemedicine for stroke. *Stroke.* 1999;30:464–469.
9. Business Wire. *Specialists on Call Oversees its 10,000th tPA Administration to an Acute Stroke Patient.* vol. December 2. Business Wire; 2015. https://www.businesswire.com/news/home/20151202006018/en/Specialists-Call-Oversees-10000th-tPA-Administration-Acute.
10. Courneya PT, Palattao KJ, Gallagher JM. HealthPartners' online clinic for simple conditions delivers savings of $88 per episode and high patient approval. *Health Aff (Millwood).* 2013;32:385–392.
11. Daschle T, Dorsey ER. The return of the house call. *Ann Intern Med.* 2015;162:587–588.
12. McConnochie KM, et al. Telemedicine reduces absence resulting from illness in urban child care: evaluation of an innovation. *Pediatrics.* 2005;115:1273–1282.
13. Uscher-Pines L, Mehrotra A. Analysis of Teladoc use seems to indicate expanded access to care for patients without prior connection to a provider. *Health Aff (Millwood).* 2014;33:258–264.

14. Thomas L, Capistrant G. *State Telemedicine Gaps Analysis Coverage and Reimbursement.* mTelehealth; 2016. https://mtelehealth.com/state-telemedicine-gaps-analysis-coverage-reimbursement/.

15. Neufeld JD, Doarn CR. Telemedicine spending by Medicare: a snapshot from 2012. *Telemed J E Health.* 2015;21:686–693.

16. AMA Online. *CARES Act: AMA COVID-19 Pandemic Telehealth Fact Sheet.* vol. 2020. AMA online; 2020. https://www.ama-assn.org/delivering-care/public-health/cares-act-ama-covid-19-pandemic-telehealth-fact-sheet.

17. Chaudhry HJ, Robin LA, Fish EM, Polk DH, Gifford JD. Improving access and mobility—the interstate medical licensure compact. *N Engl J Med.* 2015;372:1581–1583.

18. Nunes D. HR 3081 TELE-MED Act of 2015. In: *114th Congress;* 2015. https://www.congress.gov/bill/114th-congress/house-bill/3081.

19. Wicklund E. *New Bill Would OK Telehealth Anywhere for 6 Months After COVID-19 Emergency.* vol. 2020. mHealth Intelligence; 2020. https://mhealthintelligence.com/news/new-bill-would-ok-telehealth-anywhere-for-6-months-after-covid-19-emergency.

20. Pearl R. Kaiser Permanente northern California: current experiences with internet, mobile, and video technologies. *Health Aff (Millwood).* 2014;33:251–257.

21. Center, M.A.C. *Unpublished Virtual Visit Data.* MDACC; 2020.

22. Mobasheri MH, Johnston M, Syed UM, King D, Darzi A. The uses of smartphones and tablet devices in surgery: a systematic review of the literature. *Surgery.* 2015;158:1352–1371.

23. Dorsey ER, Glidden AM, Holloway MR, Birbeck GL, Schwamm LH. Teleneurology and mobile technologies: the future of neurological care. *Nat Rev Neurol.* 2018;14:285–297.

24. Jonker LT, Haveman ME, de Bock GH, van Leeuwen BL, Lahr MMH. Feasibility of perioperative eHealth interventions for older surgical patients: a systematic review. *J Am Med Dir Assoc.* 2020.

25. Gladwell M. *The Tipping Point: How Little Things Can Make a Big Difference.* Boston: Little Brown; 2000.

26. Moses 3rd H, et al. The anatomy of medical research: US and international comparisons. *JAMA.* 2015;313:174–189.

27. Businesswire. *Venture Capital Funding in Digital Health Sector Reaches $8.9B in 2019.* Businesswire; 2020. https://www.businesswire.com/news/home/20200115005574/en/Venture-Capital-Funding-Digital-Health-Sector-Reaches#:~:text=Venture%20Capital%20Funding%20in%20Digital%20Health%20Sector%20Reaches%20%248.9%20Billion%20in%202019,-%2458%20billion%20has&text=Global%20venture%20capital%20(VC)%20funding,in%20698%20deals%20in%202018.

28. Group, M.C. *Q4 and Annual 2019 Digital Health (Healthcare IT) Funding and M&A Report;* 2020. https://mercomcapital.com/product/q4-annual-2019-digital-health-healthcare-it-funding-ma-report/.

29. Ray KN, Chari AV, Engberg J, Bertolet M, Mehrotra A. Disparities in time spent seeking medical care in the United States. *JAMA Intern Med.* 2015;175:1983–1986.

30. Anderson G. *Chronic Care;* 2010. https://www.rwjf.org/en/library/research/2010/01/chronic-care.html.

31. Achey MA, et al. Erratum To: Virtual house calls for Parkinson disease (Connect.Parkinson): study protocol for a randomized, controlled trial. *Trials.* 2016;17:7.

32. Cramer SC, et al. Efficacy of home-based telerehabilitation vs in-clinic therapy for adults after stroke: a randomized clinical trial. *JAMA Neurol.* 2019.

33. Espay AJ, et al. A roadmap for implementation of patient-centered digital outcome measures in Parkinson's disease obtained using mobile health technologies. *Mov Disord.* 2019;34:657–663.

34. Fisher RS, et al. Seizure diaries for clinical research and practice: limitations and future prospects. *Epilepsy Behav.* 2012;24:304–310.
35. van Oosterhout WP, et al. Validation of the web-based LUMINA questionnaire for recruiting large cohorts of migraineurs. *Cephalalgia.* 2011;31:1359–1367.
36. Lanham NS, Bockelman KJ, McCriskin BJ. Telemedicine and orthopaedic surgery: the COVID-19 pandemic and our new normal. *JBJS Rev.* 2020;8, e2000083.
37. Laskowski ER, et al. The telemedicine musculoskeletal examination. *Mayo Clin Proc.* 2020;95:1715–1731.
38. Satcher RL, et al. Telemedicine and telesurgery in cancer care: inaugural conference at MD Anderson Cancer Center. *J Surg Oncol.* 2014;110:353–359.
39. Meyer GS, Gibbons RV. House calls to the elderly—a vanishing practice among physicians. *N Engl J Med.* 1997;337:1815–1820.
40. Beck CA, et al. National randomized controlled trial of virtual house calls for Parkinson disease. *Neurology.* 2017;89:1152–1161.
41. Hampton JR, Harrison MJ, Mitchell JR, Prichard JS, Seymour C. Relative contributions of history-taking, physical examination, and laboratory investigation to diagnosis and management of medical outpatients. *Br Med J.* 1975;2:486–489.
42. Center PR. *Mobile Fact Sheet;* 2019. https://www.pewresearch.org/internet/fact-sheet/mobile/.
43. Krittanawong C, Zhang H, Wang Z, Aydar M, Kitai T. Artificial intelligence in precision cardiovascular medicine. *J Am Coll Cardiol.* 2017;69:2657–2664.
44. D'Amario D, et al. Telemedicine, artificial intelligence and humanisation of clinical pathways in heart failure management: back to the future and beyond. *Card Fail Rev.* 2020;6, e16.
45. Khoury MJ, Gwinn ML, Glasgow RE, Kramer BS. A population approach to precision medicine. *Am J Prev Med.* 2012;42:639–645.
46. Maier M, Takano T, Sapir-Pichhadze R. Changing paradigms in the management of rejection in kidney transplantation: evolving from protocol-based care to the era of P4 medicine. *Can J Kidney Health Dis.* 2017;4, 2054358116688227.

INDEX

Note: Page numbers followed by *f* indicate figures and *t* indicate tables.

A

Academic hospital rounds, classic model of, 148–149
Accreditation Council for Graduate Medical Education (ACGME), 146–147
Adam's forward bending test, 120–121
Alertness, 22, 106
Ambulatory care, 149
American Academy of Neurology (AAN), 150–151
American Academy of Sleep Medicine (AASM), 81
American Academy of Sleep Medicine's (AASM) Taskforce on Sleep Telemedicine, 81, 85
American Psychological Association Organizational Practice Committee (IOPC), 69–72
Amyotrophic lateral sclerosis (ALS), 90–94
Anterior segment exam, 36, 44
Aphasia, 23–24, 108–109
Artificial intelligence (AI), 190
Asynchronous Consultation in Movement Disorders (ACMD) program, 171–172
Asynchronous telehealth, 31–32, 41
Asynchronous virtual visits, 49
Ataxia, 23
Audio-video telemedicine, 12

B

Babinski reflex, 112–113
Billing, tele-neuropsychology, 73–74
Boston Naming Test, 64
Broca's aphasia, 108–109
Burning building scenario, 12–13

C

Centers for Medicare and Medicaid Services (CMS), 183–184
Center to Center (C2C) model, 81

Center to Center Movement Disorders Training Program, 175
Center to Home (C2H) model, 81
Change management, 130–131, 135–136, 140–141
Clinical care, of teleneurology, 166–167
Cognitive behavioral therapy (CBT), 85
Color vision, 42
Commitment to cooperative growth, 127, 141–142
Communication, 5–6, 11, 14
Consent form, tele-neuropsychology, 69–72
Consultation exception, 158–159
Consultations, virtual epilepsy care, 26–27
Consumer sleep technologies (CSTs), 86
Coordination, 113–114
Coronavirus Aid, Relief, and Economic Security Act (CARES Act), 48, 61
Coronavirus disease 2019 (COVID-19) pandemic, 1, 3–4
    HM (*see* Houston Methodist (HM))
    movement disorders, 49–51, 54
    neurology, 94–95
    neuromuscular disease, 95–99
    spine (*see* Neurospine care telemedicine)
    virtual epilepsy care, 25, 27
Coronavirus Preparedness and Response Supplemental Appropriations Act 2020, 183–184
Counseling, neuro-ophthalmology evaluation, 44
Cranial nerve (CN) exam, 109–111, 109–110*t*
Cranial nerve III palsy, 111
Cranial nerve VI palsy, 111

D

Deep brain stimulation (DBS), 48–49, 168
Disability Adjusted Life Year (DALYs), 165–166

Dysarthria, 24
Dysdiadochokinesia, 114
Dysmetria, 27, 114

E
eHealth, 190–191
Electroencephalography (EEG), 168–169
    virtual epilepsy care, 27–28
Electronic health record (EHR), 147
Electronic medical records (EMRs), 17–18,
    50–51
Electronic seizure diary, 27–28
Emergency department (ED), 125, 129
Emergency medical services (EMS), 125
Endorsement, 158–159
Epilepsy, 168–169
    management (*see*Virtual epilepsy care)
Equal Access to Care Act, 184
e-visits, 162
Expressive aphasia, 108–109
Extraocular motor movement, 43–44
Extraocular movements, 22
Eye alignment, 43–44
Eye Handbook, 33, 35*f*
Eyelids, 36

F
Follow-up, virtual epilepsy care, 28
ForSee home monitoring device, 37
Fraud and abuse, 163, 163*t*
Full licensure, 158–159
Fundus exam, 36–37

G
Gaze, 22
General neurosurgery exam
    coordination, 113–114
    cranial nerve exam, 109–111
    introductory interview questions, 105–106
    mental status, 106–109
    sensory exam, 113
    strength exam, 111–112
Glasgow coma scale (GCS), 107–108, 107*t*
    troubleshooting, 108
Global Burden of Diseases (GBD), 165–166
Graduate medical education (GME),
    145–153
Gramado Declaration, 169

H
Health care professional, fiduciary role of,
    127
Health care strategy, 135–136, 141
Health Insurance Portability and
    Accountability Act (HIPPA), 12–13,
    117–118
Home monitoring, of ophthalmologic
    exam, 37
Houston Methodist (HM)
    communication, 5–6
    patient feedback, 6–7
    physician feedback, 7–10
    training, 4–5
    virtual foundation, 1–3
    virtual urgent care, 6
Hub-and-spoke model of stroke care,
    147–148
Huntington's disease (HD), 168
Hybrid telemedicine model, of
    ophthalmologic exam, 37

I
Information and communication
    technologies (ICTs), 165
In-home tele-neuropsychology visits, 69,
    70–71*t*
Insomnia, 83
International Classification of Health
    Interventions, 167
International Movement Disorders Society
    (MDS), 50
International Parkinson's Disease and
    Movement Disorder Society,
    174–175
International telestroke networks, 166–167
Interstate compacts (ICs), 74
Interstate Medical Licensure Compact,
    158–159
Intraocular pressure (IOP), 36, 43–44
Introductory interview questions,
    105–106

K
Kaiser Permanente of Northern California,
    184
Kalamazoo Consensus Statement, 14, 14*t*

L

Language, 23–24, 108, 108*t*
Level of consciousness, 107–108
Licensure, of telehealth, 158–159
Live videoconferencing, 156
Long-distance communication, 11

M

Machine learning (ML) techniques, 190
Mayo Clinic, 13
MDS Telemedicine Study Group, 50
"Medical care anywhere", 191
Medicare 2020 COVID-19 expansion,
    160–164, 161*f*
Mental health, during COVID-19
    pandemic, 57–59
Mental status, 106–109
Mobile Health (mHealth), 158
Motor exam, 22–23
Movement disorders, 47
    COVID-19 pandemic, 49–51
    software selection process, 50–51, 51*f*
    virtual visits, 49
Mutual recognition, 158–159

N

Narcolepsy, 84
National Institute of Health Stroke Scale
    (NIHSS), 21–24, 22*t*
National licensure, 158–159
Needs assessment, 127–128, 141
Neglect, evaluation of, 24
Neurological disorders, burden of,
    165–166
Neurology, 89–90
    COVID-19 era, 94–95
    system of care, 125–126
Neuromuscular disease, 90–94
    COVID-19 era, 95–99
Neuro-ophthalmology evaluation
    previsit preparation, 39–41
    virtual visit
        history, 41–42
        management, 44
        physical exam, 42–44
Neuropsychological reports, 72–73
Neuropsychology (NP), 61

Neurospine care telemedicine
    diagnosis, 120–121, 121*t*
    evaluation/examination, 118–120, 119*t*
    limits, 122
    treatment, 121–122
    visit, 118
Neurosurgery. *See* General neurosurgery
    exam
Nocturnal Artificial Light exposure (NLE),
    81–82
Nonverbal behaviors, 15, 15*t*
North American Neuro-Ophthalmology
    Society, 44
Notal Vision, 37

O

Ocular motility, 36
Ophthalmologic exam
    anterior segment, 36
    external exam, 36
    fundus/retina, 36–37
    home monitoring, 37
    hybrid telemedicine model, 37
    intraocular pressure, 36
    ocular motility, 36
    patient selection, 31
    pupils, 35
    scheduling visits, 31–32
    software and hardware technology
        solutions, 32
    traditional exam, 32–33
    visual acuity, 33–34
    visual field, 36
Orientation, 106
OSA, 83

P

PAP therapy, 85–86
Parasomnias, 84
ParkinsonNet model, 170
Parkinson's disease (PD), 47–48, 168
Parkinson Study Group (PSG), 48–49
Patient feedback, Houston Methodist
    (HM), 6–7
Patient satisfaction, 63
Payment, for medical services, 160–164
Physical exam, of neuro-ophthalmology
    evaluation, 42–44

Physician burnout, 134, 136
Physician feedback, Houston Methodist (HM), 7–10
Picture archiving computer system (PACS), 120
Political action committees (PACs), 164
Polysomnography (PSG), 85
Practice standards, 159–160
Predictive, personalized, preventive, and participatory (P4) medicine, 190–191
Previsit preparation, virtual epilepsy care, 26
Psychological Interjurisdictional Compact (PSYPACT), 74–75

R

Radio News Magazine, 11
Real Time Audio-Video Communication, 156
Receptive aphasia, 109
Reciprocity agreement, 158–159
Reimbursement, 160, 162, 181, 183–186
Remote mental health, during COVID-19 pandemic, 57–59
Remote patient monitoring (RPM), 156–158, 162
Remote telecommunication, 108, 114
Residency programs
  academics, 149–151
  clinical duties, 147–149
Resistance, of stakeholders, 130–131, 142
Retina exam, 36–37

S

Sensory exam, 23, 113
Sleep apnea, 83, 85
Sleep telemedicine
  diagnostic approaches, 81–85
  follow-up approaches, 85–86
  technical provisions, 81, 82t
  treatment approaches, 85
Software selection process, 50–51, 51f
Special licensure, 158–159
Speech, 23–24, 108–109
Stakeholder engagement, 129, 131
State licensure, 184
St. Elizabeth System of Hospitals (StESH), 127–128, 136–137

Store and forward method, 92, 156
Strength exam, 111–112
Synchronous telemedicine, 31–32, 40–41
Synchronous virtual visits, 49
System of care
  cases, 127–128, 131–133, 136–139
  core values, 127
  definition, 125
  spoke and hub arrangement, 126
  stakeholders, 129
System-wide adoption, 136–139

T

Taskforce on Telehealth Policy, 163
Telecommunication tools, 181
Telegeria, 169–170
Telehealth/telemedicine, 57, 61–62
  academics, 149–151
  administrative, 152–153
  advocacy role, 163–164
  amyotrophic lateral sclerosis (ALS), 90–94
  basic services/modalities, 156, 157f
  chronic conditions, 187–188
  clinical duties in residency, 147–149
  clinical epilepsy, evaluation of (*see* Virtual epilepsy care)
  COVID-19 crisis, 183–184
  definition, 89
  emerging new trends, 186, 187t
  factors limiting adoption, 181, 182t
  licensure, 158–159
  medical/legal topics, 158
  Medicare, 160–164
  neurology, 89–90
    COVID-19 era, 94–95
  neuromuscular disease, 90–94
    COVID-19 era, 95–99
  neuro-ophthalmology (*see* Neuro-ophthalmology evaluation)
  ophthalmology (*see* Ophthalmologic exam)
  payment, 160–164
  practice standards, 159–160
  research, 151–152
  spine (*see* Neurospine care telemedicine)
  strength, 126
  stroke (*see* Telestroke)

teaching faculty perspective, 146–153
trainee perspective, 145
virtual visit, 13–16
    technical aspects, 16–19
Telemedicine Pilot Project for Integrative
    Stroke Care (TEMPiS), 166–167
Telemedicine Study Group of the
    International Parkinson's disease,
    173–174
Teleneurology
    education, 174–175
    Humanitarian crisis, 172–174
    movement disorders (see Movement
        disorders)
    PD (see Parkinson's disease (PD))
    preventive medicine, 169–170
    service line, after-hour calls, 132, 132f
    underserved areas, 170–172
Tele-neuropsychology (tele-NP), 61
    advantages and disadvantages, 62, 62t
    billing, 73–74
    consent form, 69–72
    future of, 75–76
    in-home visits, 69, 70–71t
    interstate practice, 74–75
    models, 66–68
    patient satisfaction, 63
    reports, 72–73
    research, 64–66
        adults, 64–65
        pediatrics, 66
Tele-psychology
    COVID-19 pandemic, 57–59
Telestroke
    evaluation, 21–24
    program, 183
    system of care, 126
Tele-technology, 61

Temporary Reciprocity to Ensure Access to
    Treatment (TREAT) Act, 184
Training, 4–5, 145

U
UTHealth TeleMed platform, 32, 34f

V
Venture capital funding, 163, 186
Veterans Affairs Neuropathy Scale (VANS),
    97–98, 97f
Veterans E-Health and Telemedicine
    Support (VETS) Act, 184
Videoconferencing administration, 64–65, 65t
Video visit checklist, 19t
Virtual check-ins, 162
Virtual epilepsy care
    COVID-19 pandemic, 25, 27
    evaluation and management, 27–28
    history and physical examination, 26–27
    opportunities, 25–26
    previsit preparation, 26
Virtual medicine, 7
Virtual urgent care, Houston Methodist
    (HM), 6, 7f
Virtual visits, 13–16
    movement disorders, 49
    neuro-ophthalmology evaluation
        history, 41–42
        management, 44
        physical exam, 42–44
    neurospine care telemedicine, 118
    technical aspects, 16–19
Visual acuity, 33–34, 42
Visual fields, 22, 36, 42–43

W
Wernicke's aphasia, 109